Understanding Girls

with

Attention Deficit

Hyperactivity Disorder

Kathleen G. Nadeau, Ph.D.
Ellen B. Littman, Ph.D.
Patricia O. Quinn, M.D.

Advantage Books
Silver Spring, MD
1999

Advantage Books

Library of Congress Cataloging-in-Publication Data

Nadeau, Kathleen G.
    Understanding Girls with AD/HD / Kathleen Nadeau,
    Ellen Littman, Patricia Quinn
        p.   cm.
    ISBN O-9660366-5-4
    1. Attention-deficit-disordered children.
    2. Girls—Mental health.
    3. Hyperactive Children.
    I. Littman, Ellen, 1954-
    II. Quinn Patricia O.
    III. Title.
    RJ506.H9N333   1999
    618.92'8589'0082—dc21

Case histories in this book are either composites of several patients' histories or
are stories submitted by actual patients or their families. Identities have been
changed to protect patient confidentiality.

The term AD/HD is used in this book in order to conform with current
nomenclature. It is intended to include all aspects of the disorder, including
non-hyperactive type, and is at times interchangeable with the terms ADD,
ADHD, or ADD-H.

Published by
Advantage Books
1001 Spring Street, Suite 206
Silver Spring, MD 20910

10 9 8 7 6 5
Printed in the U. S. A.

Foreword

In the Spring of 1998, after attending two separate gatherings, it became apparent to me that, recently, we have entered an exciting new era for women and girls with AD/HD. The first of these gatherings was a talk given at Eastern Michigan University by Carol Gilligan, Ph.D., in which she explained her concept of the "resonance chamber," the space created by women speaking together and giving voice to their own experiences. This pioneering psychologist and author of the groundbreaking book, *In a Different Voice*, explained that when women and girls come together to speak the truth of their own experiences, they create a chamber where women's voices amplify and validate one another. Instead of hearing their truths come back to them in distorted ways, as is common in the general culture, they begin to hear their own truths in a clear, strong way. Instead of remaining silent and pretending "not to know what they know" about themselves, their own voices grow more confident, forever changing them personally, as well as affecting the larger political system in which they live.

The second occasion took place only the next day at the *Annual Conference of The National Attention Deficit Disorder Association* in Washington, D.C., where I led the first ever *Woman's Forum for Women with AD/HD*. The forum brought together a large group of women with AD/HD from around the world that was gathering to speak to each other about their personal experiences. Among them were housewives, writers, doctors, even specialists in the field of AD/HD, though no one was allowed to speak as a specialist or an "expert." Although I had not known of Gilligan's "resonance chamber" while I was planning this gathering, I saw clearly that this group of women demonstrated what Gilligan had

iii

expressed. These women with AD/HD had not come to hear about AD/HD as a physiological or chemical disorder. They had not gathered to be told what sort of "condition" they had. Instead, they had come to tell their own stories of living with AD/HD, to define what AD/HD meant to them, to speak out and make the vital and necessary truths of their own experience heard.

The "resonance chamber" with which these women made their voices heard is reflective of a new and exciting shift away from an older model of AD/HD, which was too often not serving women. The significance of this shift is best seen in the context of psychology as a whole, which only thirty years ago tended to describe and measure women and girls by how they differed from the yardstick of so-called "normal" or male development. In the field of AD/HD, the only description and criteria we had were formulated by observers of little boys who displayed hyperactivity. This meant that, until recently, there was no way to understand the pervasiveness of the experience and the effect of AD/HD in the lives of women and girls, since they do not display hyperactivity as commonly as boys. Instead, many tend to withdraw and internalize their difficulties. They develop anxiety, depression, or people-pleasing behaviors. If these girls typically underachieve, they also do not make waves or disrupt classes, and are easily tolerated by society. As a result, girls and women with AD/HD have grown up unnoticed and untreated.

Fortunately, since the early 90s, the focus of AD/HD has broadened beyond the model of the badly-behaved little boy to include adults and, more recently and dramatically, women and girls as well. At conferences, in groups, in seminars, through magazines and on-line affiliations, women have grown increasingly confident, comfortable, and sure of their own experiences after years of silence. As a result, the first generation of women with AD/HD has gradually emerged, to be diagnosed and treated. These women are pioneers who have fought long and hard for understanding and inclusion. It is only through them that gradually we have come to understand how women and girls experience AD/HD differently and how they have struggled for years not only with AD/HD, but also with the consequences of living undiagnosed and untreated.

We know now that the girls who did not get treated for their AD/HD until adulthood often accumulated complex emotional layers, which later needed to be revealed and repaired. As a result of the confusing experiences they had growing up and the under-achievement that commonly accompanies AD/HD in girls, these individuals saw their gifts and talents fall more and more out of reach as they grew and matured. With no adults to offer an explanatory view, they were unable to internalize, as secure children need to do, a confirming and clarifying adult voice—the voice of a mother or a caring guardian—that supplies a measure of much-needed guidance and self-acceptance for children. Unable to explore their gifts, often they became quiet and removed, and uncertain about their self-image. Finally, growing into adolescence and maturity, they found themselves unable to keep up with the subtle, but definite expectations that are woven into the social matrix of being a woman. As they became part of an intimate relationship or created a family, the cultural pressure to serve as the emotional, social, and organizational center of the social unit increased. Now, in addition to their AD/HD and their confusion, they began to feel that they had failed to meet the gender role expectations of womanhood, and they internalized a great deal of shame. Ultimately, as their shame and confusion grew, so did their sense of isolation.

What we have learned from the long and hard battles fought by these pioneers will have dramatic impact on the current generation of girls with AD/HD. Thankfully, our girls will now have this information available at an early age and will be more likely to avoid the effects of growing up unidentified, untreated, and confused about their experiences. But, we must be vigilant in assuring that we use this information wisely. The danger here is that we might begin to pathologize our daughters—to define them in terms of symptoms, treatments, or an impersonal physiological and chemical "disorder" by which, if we are not careful, our girls will begin to conceptualize and see themselves.

If we are to succeed, it is important not to lose sight of our goal. We want not only to treat AD/HD, but to treat it in such a way that encourages our girls to develop their gifts, to learn to make good choices, to build a strong self-image, and to speak with assured voices. We must remember that the point of teaching our daughters how to manage AD/HD and its symptoms is not simply to make their lives perfectly organized and trouble-free. This unreasonable and counterproductive goal will teach them only to focus on their weaknesses and to lose sight of their strengths. The point, therefore, is to show our daughters how to manage their symptoms with the aims of becoming more fully themselves and of leading fulfilling and happy lives. This means that as challenging and sometimes discouraging as living with AD/HD can be, our daughters must not see their differences as cause for shame, which will send them back into hiding, into the quiet and removed place from which we had hoped to free them. Only if we teach them to value and use their differences can we finally empower them, rather than pathologize them.

In light of this, I would like to suggest one of the major strengths that I believe girls with AD/HD will, with some help and guidance, be able to claim and use as they mature into adolescence and adulthood. In her book *Reviving Ophelia*, Mary Pipher, Ph.D. emphasizes the danger of conforming to certain idealized and unhealthy gender roles to which all girls are subject in our culture. To protect themselves from this threat, as Pipher points out, they must find a way to hold on to their individuality. It is in facing this dilemma, I believe, that our girls with AD/HD, who find it more difficult to conform, actually can be at an advantage. As Pipher says, those girls who can conform, will, while those who cannot will need us to provide a "protected space" for them in which they can grow and develop. In this way, instead of being lost to mass cultural forces that often destroy them, our daughters will emerge from adolescence as whole, unique, strong women.

If they are to thrive as nonconformists, it will be important for our girls to have role models of strong women who may or may not have had AD/HD themselves. Some examples of such nonconformists that Pipher offers are Maya Angelou, Eleanor Roosevelt, Margaret Mead, and Madame Curie, all of whom developed their uniqueness and gifts, in some ways, because of their inability to conform. These women, Pipher explains, ultimately thrived because they had somehow internalized a confirming voice—the voice of a mother or caring role model. This voice gave them the guidance and permission to be who they were and to occupy their own internal protected spaces apart from the culture that had no room for them. In their protected spaces, as Pipher points out, these women were able to fall in love with ideas, to dedicate themselves to special passions, and to retreat to secret places where they could dream for hours. All of these are behavior patterns that finally led to their successes and which, I would like to emphasize, resemble some of the behavior patterns of many of our girls with AD/HD.

Too often, however, when parents see their daughters not fitting in, they become alarmed, and unwittingly send their girls the message that their differences are a weakness and a cause for shame. But this is often a counterproductive response. Instead, it is essential that we provide for our daughters a confirming and supportive voice, which then they can internalize. This will allow them to value themselves as gifted non-conformists and, as such, give them license to dream.

The collective voices that create books such as *Understanding Girls with AD/HD* help give us the power to provide just the sort of protected space that is necessary if we are to shelter and value the differences in our daughters, and if we are ultimately to teach our daughters to value themselves. And it is in this space of "resonance," to borrow Gilligan's words again, that we can and must continue to speak our own truth for ourselves, for our daughters, our clients and our students. Only by speaking out with strong voices and by valuing our own differences as women can we ultimately serve as the role models that our daughters will need. In this way, we can become partners with them on their journey towards authentic and full lives. In this way, we and our daughters can have the courage to speak and to "know what we know."

Sari Solden, M. S., LMFT
Author of *Women with Attention Deficit Disorder*
Ann Arbor, June, 1999

Table of Contents

Dedication

We would like to dedicate this book to all the girls and women that we have known over the years who have taught us to better understand what it is to be a girl with Attention Deficit/Hyperactivity Disorder. We are only at the beginning. There is much to learn. In partnership with them, we can move forward together, expanding and improving our understanding, making it more likely that future girls with AD/HD will grow up to lead authentic, self-affirming lives.

— *Kathleen G. Nadeau, Ph.D.*
Ellen B. Littman, Ph.D.
Patricia O. Quinn, M.D.

Acknowledgements

We would like to acknowledge the help of many people in the creation of this book. A special thanks to Wendy Sharp, research social worker at the NIH, for her early input regarding current research on gender issues in AD/HD. Thanks also go to Dr. Deborah Fisher who generously gave us feedback and input as we developed the initial version of our Girls AD/HD Self-Report Questionnaire. Thanks to Sari Solden, pioneer in the field of women's AD/HD issues, who helped us to become more aware of the range of issues that these women had faced growing up as girls with undiagnosed AD/HD. Our appreciation also must be expressed to the many women and mothers who responded to our request for stories from families of girls with AD/HD. Their generosity has made the creation of this book very much a group effort. Likewise, we want to acknowledge the women who have allowed their stories and their poetry to be used in our book. We believe that their contributions will be very helpful to the generations of girls growing up today. Thanks to Dr. Barbara Ingersoll for her valuable feedback and encouragement, and to Thom Hartmann, who generously shared his experiences in raising a daughter with AD/HD. And, finally, an immeasurable thank you to Langdon Nadeau, whose energy, creativity and valiant struggles inspired her mother to initiate the writing of this book.

Contributors

Kathleen G. Nadeau, Ph.D., is a licensed clinical psychologist and the author of numerous books on Attention Deficit Disorder who gives lectures and workshops on AD/HD nationally. She earned her doctorate in clinical psychology from the University of Florida in 1971 and has lived and worked in the Washington, D.C. area throughout her professional life. Dr. Nadeau is the Director of Chesapeake Psychological Services of Maryland, a clinic providing a broad range of diagnostic and treatment services for individuals with AD/HD.

Ellen B. Littman, Ph.D. is a licensed clinical psychologist, educated and trained at Brown and Yale Universities, and at the Albert Einstein College of Medicine. Involved in the AD/HD field for over 15 years, she teaches, lectures, provides inservice training, and conducts research on gender issues in AD/HD. Dr. Littman's private practice in Mount Kisco, NY specializes in individual, couples, and group treatment for AD/HD adults.

Patricia O. Quinn, M.D. is a developmental pediatrician in the Washington, D.C. area. A graduate of the Georgetown University Medical School, she specializes in child development and psychopharmacology. Dr. Quinn has worked for over 25 years in the areas of AD/HD and learning disabilities. She gives workshops nationwide and has published widely in these fields.

Chapter One

What I Wish They Had Understood When I Was a Girl

We understand far too little about girls with AD/HD. How are they similar to boys with AD/HD? How do they differ? How many girls are there with AD/HD? Field studies of children with AD/HD suggest that the proportion of girls in the general population is significantly higher (3:1) than the proportion of girls who are referred to clinics (from 9:1 to 6:1) (Szatmari et al., 1989; American Psychiatric Association, 1987). Informal reports suggest that the percentage of women seeking treatment for AD/HD is significantly higher than the percentage of girls who are treated for AD/HD. A recent study of parents of children diagnosed with AD/HD revealed that the number of mothers and fathers reporting significant AD/HD symptoms in themselves was equal, lending more evidence to a growing suspicion that earlier studies have greatly underestimated the number of females with AD/HD (Walker, 1999). These various studies all strongly suggest that girls are being under-diagnosed. One of the central missions of this book is to understand why this may be the case. What has prevented many young girls from being identified and helped?

Most women with AD/HD were only able to seek help as adults, after many years of feeling frustrated, inadequate, and misunderstood. Our hope is that girls growing up today with AD/HD can avoid this fate. Early diagnosis and treatment is critical to allow girls to reach their full potential as women.

In this chapter, women with AD/HD tell their unique stories about growing up without understanding the cause of their struggles. These are stories of thwarted efforts to perform academically, of shame, self-blame, and feelings of low self-worth. The women describe their forgetfulness, and the messiness and chaos of their desks, bedrooms, and schoolbags. They talk about the social difficulties that led them to feel like misfits, never knowing quite how to find acceptance in the all-important social world of girls. We have asked these women to look back on their childhoods and tell us what they wish their parents and teachers had known. They offer a unique gift—insight into the life of a girl with AD/HD from the perspective and understanding of an adult.

I Wish My Mother Had Known

By Mary H.

I wish my mother had known
that I was actually very smart.
I wish my mother had known
that I needed more attention.

*I wish my mother had known
that I went to school every day as a little girl,
in fear and dread
at the prospect of being shamed
and humiliated in class.*

*I wish my mother had known
that my low self-esteem and
lack of physical affection at home
would lead to rampant promiscuity.*

*I wish my mother had known
that someday I would have to
compete in the world,
and that being married
was not going to make me safe.*

*I wish my mother had known how desperately
I needed stimulation and attainable challenges.
(Expectations for me were very low,
so even I was surprised when I realized
that I love a challenge!)*

*I wish my mother had known
that my artistic and creative skills
were important,
and could have sustained me,
had I been encouraged to develop them.*

*I wish my mother had known
that I could not organize my room.*

*I wish my mother had known
that I had a huge curiosity about life,
but that I could not absorb it
in the context of public school.*

I wish my mother had known
that I was too sensitive and shy and embarrassed
to have my needs met.

I wish my mother had known
that I could not easily either fall asleep or wake up,
and that I had no control over that.

I wish my mother had known that being put
into the dumb classes,
in spite of my consistently high IQ tests,
was humiliating,
and caused me to not even bother to try.

I wish my mother had known
that having only one friend
was not normal and might have signaled other problems.

I wish my mother had known
that leaving the house unzipped, buttoned wrong,
or without my lunch or books, was a signal.

I wish my mother had known
what we know now.
She didn't. She did her best,
and I hope that she knows
how very much I love her.

Mary, the author of this poetic lament, outlines the very issues that we need to address. Although she directs her comments toward her mother, all of us who know girls with AD/HD should take note. There are many "Marys" sitting in today's classrooms. These are girls whose potential goes unrecognized, even when measured, as Mary's was. These are girls who go to great effort to hide in the classroom to escape the teacher's notice, whose learning style is unrecognized, whose talents are not considered relevant, and who suffer greatly as a result.

Signs of underlying AD/HD issues

Mary's wish list almost can serve as an outline for our book. She details the behaviors that should have signaled to her parents and teachers that there were underlying problems:

- School phobia or avoidance
- Low self-esteem
- High IQ and creativity, but low academic performance
- Poor organizational skills, messiness
- Sleep problems
- Shyness
- Poor social skills
- Disheveled appearance, grooming problems
- Withdrawal in the classroom

Possible solutions

Mary describes the unwitting assumptions that allowed both her parents and teachers to overlook and undervalue her talents and abilities; and she relates not only the causes, but the possible solutions that could have helped her overcome her limitations:

- Understanding of her struggles

- Attention and affection to offset daily assaults to her self-esteem

- Affirmation and encouragement of her creativity

- Recognition of her high IQ

- Acknowledgment of her need for a different learning environment

- Appropriate stimulation and challenges

- Help with structure and organization

- Help with sleep problems

- Support to develop assertiveness skills

- Recognition of social difficulties and help in learning social skills

Women without AD/HD—Challenged to understand

Mary also illustrates the problem that so often occurs when a mother without AD/HD raises a daughter with AD/HD—a great difficulty in accepting or understanding why their daughter is forgetful, disorganized, and unfocused. For parents and teachers who have not experienced similar dilemmas themselves, understanding the workings of a brain with AD/HD takes a great deal of imagination, empathy, and determined efforts to learn complex information about neuro-cognitive functioning.

Patterns in boys are easier to recognize

The majority of our classroom teachers, like Mary's mother, also a former teacher, are women without AD/HD: women who were comfortable in the classroom environment as girls, who elected to remain in that environment as adults; women who are able to plan, to organize, and to attend to details. Teachers can, perhaps, more readily recognize the "differentness" of boys with AD/HD. Their impulsivity, high activity level, and disruptiveness are easy to detect, and they create classroom dilemmas any teacher would be eager to minimize. Thus, boys are most often referred for diagnosis and treatment.

Patterns in girls are less understood

Teachers without AD/HD may have greater difficulty accepting and appreciating as AD/HD symptoms the feelings and behaviors more typical of girls with AD/HD. These include patterns such as talkativeness, social withdrawal, a tendency to miss or misunderstand directions, messiness, disorganization, test anxiety, late or missing assignments, and forgetfulness. Even an intense, anxious, hyper-focus on schoolwork may signal a girl with AD/HD who is frantically attempting to compensate for her difficulties.

That's not ladylike!

Research shows that mothers of girls with AD/HD tend to be more critical of their daughters than are mothers of sons with AD/HD (Barkley, 1991). Might this be true for teachers as well? Are they less tolerant or supportive of girls who demonstrate AD/HD patterns? We need more research, but anecdotal evidence suggests that girls who forget their lunch money, lose their homework, or seem unmotivated in class are more likely to be admonished than to be referred for evaluation. Our goal in this book is to alert parents, teachers, and the professional community about the more subtle signs of

AD/HD in girls, and to focus on the special needs of these girls both within and outside the classroom.

Women with AD/HD—A key to understanding girls

More research on gender issues in AD/HD is needed. One of the critical questions is how we can develop more appropriate diagnostic criteria. Adult women with recently diagnosed AD/HD may hold the answers, and should be considered a vast, untapped reservoir of information concerning girls with AD/HD. This rich resource can provide invaluable direction for developing better guidelines to identify girls with AD/HD today. By asking women with AD/HD about their childhood experiences, we can learn first-hand about what it is like to be a girl growing up with AD/HD. By listening to their collective voices, we can develop critical insights that will allow us to diagnose and treat our current generation of girls with AD/HD.

To better understand just how important diagnosis and treatment is, let's look at the stories of three women, now middle-aged, who were bright children with tremendous potential, but who weren't diagnosed or treated until adulthood. Each of them has paid a high price for this delayed diagnosis.

Nora's story

Nora was an active, vivacious, argumentative, and willful girl, whose home life was characterized by a series of eruptions. She recalls intense arguments with her father, who battled with her verbally and, at times, physically. He regularly called her "stupid," occasionally even throwing things at her. These violent interactions occurred when Nora voiced her strong opinions, typically in direct, confrontational disagreement with her father.

When Nora was nine years old, the family entered treatment to reduce the conflict level at home. The treatment, however, focused on the family depression and dysfunction, not on Nora's behavior patterns. Her need for structure and support at home and school went unrecognized. Nora began drug experimentation at an early age, a common pattern for girls with AD/HD. (In fact, a recent study (Biederman et al., 1999) indicates that up to 4% of girls with AD/HD have experimented with drugs as early as age eleven, with a much higher percentage of adolescent girls with AD/HD becoming involved in substance abuse.) Nora hardly studied and earned mediocre grades. Despite her poor study habits, Nora's high IQ enabled her to pass from one grade to the next, eventually graduating from high school at the age of eighteen.

After graduation, Nora remained at home, attending a local college. Although she dreamed of becoming a teacher or a lawyer, her spotty, inconsistent performance continued. Midway through college she dropped out of school to marry Charles, a young man who was also quite intelligent, but different from Nora in other ways.

Charles was highly structured, driven, and bordering on the obsessional in his need for order and predictability. At first, his rigid patterns appealed to Nora, who had sorely lacked structure while growing up. But his need to control her soon grew oppressive, and finally intolerable. After giving birth to two sons, both of whom were later diagnosed with AD/HD, Nora ended what had ultimately become a destructive, combative marriage.

In her late twenties, she found herself under-employed, and barely able to support herself and her two sons, despite financial assistance from her parents and ex-husband. She was overwhelmed by the responsibilities of work, the demands of single-parenting two very challenging children, and the need to somehow find time to manage her budget and her household. With her life coming apart at the seams, Nora entered treatment for AD/HD and depression.

Six years later, Nora has rearranged her life into one that is more AD/HD-friendly. She now shares custody of her two sons, rather than struggling alone as their primary parent. She has advocated fiercely for her sons in the school system, and is primarily responsible for the special educational supports they are given—supports she needed, but never received during her own school years. She has learned techniques to better manage her household and her budget. Nora has become an active advocate for herself and for others with disabilities at her workplace, and has received two promotions on the job. She has developed excellent computer skills and is thinking of returning to college to complete her education. We can only wonder how much of the chaos and underachievement that has marked her life could have been avoided had her AD/HD been properly treated throughout childhood.

Gloria's story

Gloria's story is very different from Nora's, and gives a good illustration of the range of patterns seen in females with AD/HD. Gloria grew up in a structured, middle-class home, attended private schools, and enjoyed the love of her parents and siblings. Although her childhood years were much calmer than Nora's, her strongest recollection was a feeling that she constantly disappointed her parents, failing to live up to their expectations.

At age 16, Gloria impulsively dropped out of school and left home. Moving hundreds of miles away, she suddenly launched herself into independence without the experience or job skills to succeed. Gloria recalls feeling confused and puzzled, wondering why she was throwing away her dreams and goals by rushing into this ill-planned venture.

In response to her self-defeating, impulsive actions, Gloria became frightened, mistrustful of herself, and of her actions that seemed so at odds with what was socially acceptable. Like many other females with AD/HD who have little self-esteem or reason to believe in themselves, Gloria consciously adopted a mask of "normalcy" and began to play a role.

She married a man who could offer her financial security and structure, and she committed herself to a life of raising children and managing a home, albeit with much difficulty, given her undiagnosed AD/HD. Seemingly competent and content with her role of wife and mother, Gloria lived for years with a sense of growing desperation while wondering if all women struggled as hard as she did to manage the daily tasks of raising children.

Gloria describes these years as "living my life on a stage, repeating my superwoman act day after day, until finally, too tired and burnt out to continue, I took off my mask and revealed my true self." In her mid-thirties her "superwoman act" collapsed. Gloria's family, who had only known the "mask," responded with dismay and disappointment. Gloria declared that she was unable to go on meeting her family's needs at such a painful cost to herself.

Her awakening came as she read a book entitled *Women*

with Attention Deficit Disorder and found her life described on every page. Finally, there was an explanation for her impulsivity, her inconsistency, her chronic lateness, her difficulty keeping an ordered home, and her abandoned hopes and dreams. Gloria received a diagnosis of AD/HD, began to take medication, and made the courageous decision, as a 38-year-old mother of four, to go to college. She and her family have together learned about AD/HD, and several of her children have been diagnosed with AD/HD as well.

Now, a few years later, she has maintained a 4.0 grade point average in college and hopes to pursue graduate study in the field of medicine. Gloria's college-age daughter is also diagnosed with AD/HD. Because she has had the enormous benefit of her mother's knowledge and understanding of AD/HD, her path will be much smoother. She has attended college, has solid self-esteem, and works actively with her mother to promote awareness of AD/HD in girls and women. The contrast between Gloria's early years and those of her daughter paint a vivid picture of the value of early diagnosis and treatment.

Elaine's story

Elaine has a different story of underachievement. Unlike Nora, who was strong-willed and fiercely argumentative, or Gloria, who successfully adopted the "mask" of the ideal wife and mother, Elaine struggled quietly throughout childhood and adulthood due to both undiagnosed AD/HD and learning disabilities.

As a girl, Elaine recalls being criticized by her mother for being "slow." Later, as a wife and mother, Elaine endured the criticism of her husband, who disliked her messiness, her inconsistency with the children, and her difficulty maintaining employment. Elaine recalls that as a girl she felt brighter than some other children, and couldn't understand why her assignments in school were so laborious for her. Significantly, though, during certain periods in her childhood, she was able to excel academically due to extra support and structure. One of these periods occurred when she was enrolled in a highly structured school in Europe where her father was temporarily assigned. A second time of academic success came in fourth grade when she received daily support from her mother. Due to her poor academic performance, the school had proposed retaining Elaine in fourth grade for another year. Elaine's mother made a special effort to help her each day so that she could progress to fifth grade along with her peers. Elaine blossomed under this individual tutoring. Unfortunately, it stopped when Elaine was successfully promoted to fifth grade. We can only speculate about the level of academic success that she might have achieved had she continued to receive this much-needed individual support.

Elaine's academic achievement remained mediocre in later grades. She recalls in ninth grade the assignment of a long-term research paper. She checked out a pile of books from the library, but not knowing how to proceed, felt paralyzed and could not write her paper. Elaine received an "F," which she recalls painfully to this day.

After high school, Elaine attended a small college for women where, despite working harder than many of her peers, she was able to earn only mediocre grades. She married shortly after graduation, but, unlike Gloria, she was unable to meet her husband's expectations as a wife and mother. Her disorganization was always an issue in her marriage. She tried to work periodically during her marriage, but usually felt inadequate. Without benefit of an AD/HD and LD diagnosis, and with little understanding of her strengths, Elaine repeatedly sought work that targeted her weaknesses. She felt that she was a failure, both at home and at work.

Her marriage ended in divorce when her two daughters were in their teens. Elaine's employment record continued to be spotty. She moved from job to job, sometimes being fired, more often leaving due to profound unhappiness. Finally, she found herself in a low-paying, part-time job assisting a nurse in a high school health clinic. This nurse, recognizing Elaine's abilities, her motivation, and her concern for the students, encouraged Elaine to study nursing.

Elaine began a course of study at the local community college, but her pattern of academic struggles soon re-emerged. She felt overwhelmed, despite her best efforts. A counselor suggested that she seek an evaluation of her learning problems. Testing revealed that Elaine had both AD/HD and learning disabilities involving a weakness in verbal memory and written language.

Due to the great demand for memorization in the study of nursing, and in light of the pattern of strengths and weaknesses discovered through the psycho-educational testing, Elaine was encouraged to shift her focus of studies to social work. Social work, like nursing, was a good match for her personality type, but would allow her to use her strengths rather than her weaknesses.

Today, Elaine has been in treatment for AD/HD for several years. With the benefit of a good career match, medication, tutoring, and supportive therapy, she has completed her master's degree in social work, earning A's on her graduate papers. Elaine is highly regarded at work and has a promising future despite her very late start. Once again, we must ask ourselves: what could Elaine have attained, and how many years of failure could she have avoided, if she had received needed assistance as a girl?

The healing power of understanding

A recent research project looked at women with AD/HD who have been diagnosed as adults (Rucklidge & Kaplan, 1998). One of the important findings of this study is that the diagnosis alone, even without treatment, seems to have a very beneficial effect for these women. The diagnosis of AD/HD gives them an explanation and a structure they can use to reframe and redefine their long history of difficulties. "I'm not losing my head, or going crazy; there is a reason I'm like this. . . relief, a lot of relief is what I feel." "When I was diagnosed and labeled, it was one of the most cathartic points in my life." "It made such an impact on how I felt about me!" "It was such a relief to get a name for it; it was so freeing!"

Just knowing and understanding the diagnosis began to change these women's feelings and even to help them change their behavior. "I am now aware that I switch off and don't listen, so I take precautions." "I now think of consequences and outcomes; I'm not as impulsive." "I'm more realistic now with my expectations of myself."

The diagnosis also helped reduce the destructive self-blame these women had lived with all of their lives. "The diagnosis helped me understand why I didn't do well in school, changing the blame from laziness to a medical condition." "If I'd known about AD/HD at the time I wouldn't have blamed myself so much; if someone could have helped me I would have had more control." "I now accept that it wasn't my fault in the past, it was circumstances." "I am more understanding, kinder to myself now." "I allow myself to make mistakes, not berate myself anymore, as I did as a child."

With the benefit of a diagnosis, and the changing perceptions of themselves that this brings, these women also report changes in their perceptions of their own children. "I don't want my kids to feel as I did as a kid." "I am much kinder and more understanding of my children," "I felt strongly that it wouldn't happen to my own child. I knew how it felt . . . I feel very strongly about reducing humiliation for my kids."

Understandably, along with all of the positive effects of diagnosis, these women also experience intense regret. "I hated being a child—now that I can see there is help, I would like to grow up again. I feel a lot of regret." "I wonder if I could have done better. Maybe I could have been a doctor." "It makes me think: wouldn't it have been nice to have known as a child, to get help?"

In closing

The stories of these women illustrate the enormous cost of having AD/HD undiagnosed and untreated in childhood. But these three women are among the fortunate ones who have finally had the benefit of diagnosis and treatment. There are many others who continue to struggle, blaming themselves for their failures, and unable to fulfill their potential. The gift that Elaine, Nora, and Gloria offer us is the understanding that is needed to identify and help the girls and women with AD/HD who have yet to be diagnosed.

Chapter Two

What's Different About Girls with AD/HD?

For many years children with AD/HD were called "hyperactive." Hyperactivity was thought to be the most important element among the list of traits associated with the disorder. Then, in 1968, the official diagnostic symptom list, published by the American Psychiatric Association in their Diagnostic and Statistical Manual, Second Edition (DSM II), was modified to include inattention and impulsivity. However, despite this change, the checklists commonly used by schools, pediatricians, and psychologists to identify children with AD/HD continue to emphasize hyperactive/impulsive behavior—patterns more typical of boys. Because girls are more likely to be inattentive and forgetful than hyperactive, these checklists often lead parents and professionals to overlook girls with attentional problems.

A product of its history

AD/HD, as it is defined today, is a product of its history, and new, non-gender-biased viewpoints are slow to develop. This is not a conspiracy to exclude girls. In part, male AD/HD patterns may be overemphasized because they are easier to observe. Girls, through biology and socialization, tend to be less active, more compliant, and less aggressive (Gaub & Carlson, 1997). Girls who are distracted, disorganized, quiet day dreamers receive less attention from parents and teachers than do boys who are more active, disruptive, and defiant. It is the squeaky wheel that gets the grease! A wake-up call is in order to sensitize clinicians, parents, and teachers to the more subtle behaviors indicative of AD/HD in girls. As long as we continue to focus on more noticeable "boy behaviors" we will under-diagnose inattentive girls, leaving them to struggle with low self-esteem and chronic academic under-achievement.

Diagnostic issues for girls with AD/HD

The latest version of the American Psychiatric Association's diagnostic manual (DSM-IV) recognizes three subtypes of AD/HD:

- Primarily Hyperactive/Impulsive
- Primarily Inattentive
- Combined Type (a combination of the first two types)

A recent study suggests that the first type—people with AD/HD who are purely hyperactive/impulsive without inattentive symptoms—may not, in fact, exist (Tzelepis, 1999), or may be very rare. In other words, it seems that the common denominators of AD/HD may be inattentiveness and distractibility. This is a very important distinction. If the emphasis shifts away from hyperactivity/impulsivity to inattention and distractibility, then parents, teachers, therapists, and researchers will start focusing more on factors that both boys and girls have in common. By recognizing the disorganized, non-hyperactive boys with AD/HD sitting in our nation's classrooms, our eyes can be opened to seeing girls who exhibit the same patterns.

Children without hyperactivity are more difficult to identify, however. One study (Epstein et al., 1991) reported that clinicians correctly diagnosed non-hyperactive AD/HD only about half the time. More training of teachers, parents, and professionals is needed to help them to identify these less obvious patterns. Screening instruments are needed that focus more on inattentive patterns, and that allow children to self-report less observable phenomena, such as shyness, school related anxieties, and difficulty staying focused while reading.

Consider the cases of Jason and Cara. Jason was diagnosed with AD/HD at age two. He was extremely hyperactive, defiant, slept little, and was prone to volcanic tantrums. His mother, desperate and exhausted, sought assistance from her pediatrician when she finally concluded that this wasn't a "stage," and that all of the well-intended parenting advice from friends and family didn't make a dent in his behavior.

Cara, on the other hand, was a quiet, sweet, and docile toddler. Her AD/HD was not identified until age 10, and was probably only diagnosed then because she had an observant mother, sophisticated in her knowledge about AD/HD. Cara posed no overt behavioral challenges. It was only her forget-fulness, disorganization, and difficulty in completing assign-ments in fifth grade that suggested to her mother that she might have attentional problems. Even then, it was Cara's mother, not her classroom teacher, who recognized the signs.

While Jason and Cara seem remarkably different, they are not atypical for their respective genders. The "Jasons" of this world will be noticed immediately because they create such challenges for the adults around them. It is critical that parents and teachers become sensitized enough to notice the "Caras" in our classrooms as well.

A need to study gender differences in AD/HD

In November, 1994, a meeting of many well-known AD/HD researchers was convened at the National Institutes of Health to consider AD/HD gender issues. The gathering of these medical and social scientists from across the nation reflected the initial rumblings of concern that we might be grossly un-der-diagnosing females as a result of the long-standing body of AD/HD research, which was conducted almost exclusively on boys.

Conference participants drew a number of conclusions, and developed even more hypotheses or questions for further study (Arnold, 1996). There was agreement that a higher percentage of boys with AD/HD than girls with AD/HD were referred for treatment. There was also much discussion at this NIMH Conference regarding appropriate instruments and rating scales to accurately study both males and females. It was suggested that there was a need to develop rating scales that were more sensitive to manifestations of AD/HD in girls, rather than to continue to use rating scales that focus primarily on the Hyperactive/Impulsive subtype of AD/HD.

Despite the numerous studies available that demonstrate that girls cluster more in the inattentive subtype (Gaub & Carlson, 1997; Biederman et al., 1999), most standardized teacher and parent rating scales continue to emphasize hyperactivity and impulsivity. An informal item analysis of the widely-used Conners Teachers Rating Scale—Revised (L) (Conners, 1997), conducted by the authors, found that among 59 items, 23 pertained to explain overt, observable, "external" (more typically male) behaviors including hyperactivity, impulsivity, angry outbursts, defiance, and risk-taking. Only 7 of the 59 items pertained to more "internal," less observable traits—typically more female—such as depression, timidity, anxiety, forgetfulness, or difficulty in listening.

Do girls with AD/HD struggle with different issues than boys?

Girls are biologically and neurologically different; they socialize and verbalize differently, and they are raised according to very different social expectations. In light of these well-documented and widely accepted gender differences, it would be very surprising if girls didn't face different struggles and manifest different behaviors than do boys with AD/HD. Parents, teachers, pediatricians, psychologists, and all of the other adults who work with girls with AD/HD need to become familiar with these differences in order to diagnose girls accurately and to provide treatment that is more appropriate to their special needs. (An in-depth discussion of treatment approaches for girls with AD/HD is addressed in Chapter 10.)

Different referral patterns

As long as we continue to use the current questionnaires that emphasize the "externalizing" behaviors more typical of boys (aggression, defiance, and other behavior management problems), as long as we use current DSM-IV diagnostic criteria, then many girls with AD/HD will be overlooked, or seen as pale shadows of their male AD/HD counterparts. Those girls who are referred for treatment may be only the most severely afflicted (Gaub & Carlson, 1996). Some researchers in the field of AD/HD have called for gender specific norms for diagnosing AD/HD (McGee & Feehan, 1991). However, at the present time we must rely on the current diagnostic criteria that were developed primarily through the observation of boys.

McGee and Feehan found that many girls overlooked by their teachers were identified by their parents as having many AD/HD characteristics. They speculated that parents may have been comparing their daughters to other girls, while teachers may have been comparing them to their classmates, half of whom are boys. By comparing girls to their male counterparts, teachers may tend to dismiss the less obvious signs of AD/HD in girls. Biederman and colleagues (1999) write that the problem of under-detection of girls derives from the fact that disruptive behaviors (more typical of boys) "drive clinic referrals." The issues of male-based diagnostic criteria and male-dominated clinic referral patterns may very easily lead to false conclusions about characteristics of "typical" girls with AD/HD. Issues of gender-referral bias have been raised before, but must be truly addressed before we can make more meaningful gender comparisons.

Cognitive differences

Studies of girls report contradictory findings regarding neuro-cognitive differences between girls and boys with AD/HD. An analysis of many studies of girls with AD/HD suggests that girls with AD/HD have greater intellectual impairment that boys (Gaub & Carlson, 1997). However, it has been speculated that the girls referred for evaluation of AD/HD (see the discussion of referral bias above) are those who have more school-related difficulties, due to lower IQ and/or learning disabilities, and may not be a truly representative sample of girls. In contrast, another study found that girls with AD/HD have fewer problems with "executive functioning" (organizing, planning, following through) than do boys with AD/HD (Seidman et al., 1997). And to confuse matters more, very recent study of girls with AD/HD (Biederman et al., 1999) reports no differences between girls and boys in their patterns of academic and cognitive impairments. We may not yet have a clear picture of cognitive differences and similarities between boys and girls with AD/HD because comparisons are clouded by the unavoidable influence of referral bias. What is clear, however, is that AD/HD is a significant issue for girls that can have a large, negative impact upon their academic achievement if it goes unrecognized and untreated.

Peer issues

Studies tend to demonstrate that girls with AD/HD experience more peer rejection than do boys with AD/HD (Gaub & Carlson, 1997). One such study (Brown et al., 1991) found that as girls with AD/HD get older they are rated as less popular with their peers. Another study (Berry et al., 1985) found that social rejection for girls with AD/HD began as early as preschool, where they were rejected or avoided by their peers more often than were boys with AD/HD. This makes sense when we think about some of the interpersonal traits commonly associated with AD/HD. Studies of girls' interactions show that girls, from a very early age, relate in a highly verbal, socially interactive manner. Cooperation and sensitivity to others are necessary to interact appropriately in typical girl-girl interactions. Because girls tend to be so socially interactive, we can expect that the difficulties with verbal expression and verbal control that some children with AD/HD experience will have a more negative impact on girls.

Boys relate more through shared activities rather than through verbal interaction. Competition, dominance, physical competence, exploration, risk-taking, and a high activity level are typically involved. Even in more passive activities, boys are more likely to gravitate to computer games requiring eye-hand coordination rather than to primarily verbal interactions. Boys with AD/HD who experience difficulties with verbal expression and with reading social cues will be much less affected in their activity-oriented social world. AD/HD traits such as risk taking, high activity level, and even aggression can be viewed as positive in many boy-boy interactions, but are outside the range of acceptable behavior for girls.

Tomboys with AD/HD

Some girls with AD/HD who don't fit well into the social world of girls interact more with boys, engaging in physically active, competitive, and, sometimes, risky behaviors. Viewed at "tomboys" in early years, in adolescence these girls may find acceptance by centering their social life around team sports with other athletic girls.

Hyper-social girls with AD/HD

For other girls, hyperactivity is manifested through being hyper-verbal. Such girls may adopt roles of being "silly," "crazy," or a "show-off" in their attempt to find social acceptance. In teen years, these girls may engage in more risky behaviors such as drinking, drugs, and sexual promiscuity. Attempting to compensate for their academic struggles and social differences, they may work frantically to bolster self-esteem through peer acceptance and sexuality to compensate for lower academic performance or lack of other achievements.

Shy, withdrawn girls with AD/HD

Quiet, more introverted, inattentive-type girls encounter their own types of social struggles. These girls may have problems related to shyness, timidity, and, in some cases, expressive language difficulties. They are more likely to be neglected and ignored by their peers than to experience the outright rejection and criticism experienced by some hyperactive/impulsive girls (Wheeler & Carlson, 1994). These girls may tend to withdraw socially. Feeling overwhelmed by the fast pace of verbal interaction between their female classmates, they may remove themselves at school and limit themselves to one or two friends outside of school.

Bright, hyper-focused girls with AD/HD

Those girls least likely to be identified and helped are the group of girls, typically very bright, who expend most of their energy working to compensate for their undiagnosed AD/HD. They may seem driven, or anxious, or overfocused on their studies. Their high grades mask the extreme effort that has been required to achieve them. These girls may frequently study all night to prepare for exams or to complete papers. Their hyper-focus on academics and their drive helps them to achieve, but at a very high cost. Such girls may eventually "hit the wall" when the academic demands for reading, writing, and recall increase in college and beyond. Often such girls socialize very little and don't date during high school years. They may continue to socially isolate themselves in college, unable to balance academic pursuits with social and recreational activities.

Oppositional defiant disorder/ Conduct disorder

All studies seem to be in agreement that girls with AD/ HD show significantly fewer conduct disorders or oppositional defiant disorders than do boys (Biederman et al., 1999; Arnold, 1996). This is a positive finding since children with AD/HD and behavior disorders tend to experience the most negative outcomes. However, there is a downside as well. This lower level of behavior problems seems to lead to a lower rate of teacher referral, penalizing girls who may have significant problems with inattention, but who do not draw attention to themselves through defiant behavior.

Hyperactivity

Likewise, there is general agreement across studies that girls with AD/HD are less hyperactive than are boys (Arnold, 1996). But, one question that has yet to be raised is whether hyperactivity is the same in boys and girls. For example, clinical observation suggests that hyperactivity in girls may be manifested more through hyperverbalization and emotional excitability, which are more difficult to measure and quantify than is motoric hyperactivity.

Depression

Among women who are ultimately diagnosed with AD/HD, the most common prior diagnosis they have received is that of depression. One study (Brown et al., 1989) found that girls with AD/HD had more "internalizing symptoms" such as anxiety and depression, and were more socially withdrawn than boys with AD/HD. There is evidence that symptoms of anxiety and depression become more pronounced in girls with AD/HD after puberty (Huessey, 1990). Girls with AD/HD who are shy, timid, withdrawn, and lacking in self-confidence as young girls may later develop depression. While the depression is important to recognize and to treat, it is critical that the professional community becomes aware of the possibility of underlying AD/HD in these girls and women.

A more recent study (Biederman et al., 1999) found no differences in rates of anxiety and depression in girls and boys. However, this finding may be due to the strict criteria Biederman established for rating a girl as "anxious" or "depressed." Whereas other researchers refer to moodiness and dysphoria in girls, Biederman and colleagues used much more stringent measures. To be included in that group of girls suffering from depression they had to show "marked impairment," "persistent disruption in major role functioning," or hospitalization, and to qualify as "anxious," girls in Biederman's study had to show signs of not just one, but "two or more anxiety disorders." Biederman and colleagues acknowledge in this same article that girls who are referred for treatment of AD/HD are more likely to show signs of mood and anxiety disorders than are boys.

Substance abuse/Smoking

Biederman and colleagues (1999) report a very noteworthy finding that girls with AD/HD are at a significant risk for one or more substance use disorders, in contrast to an earlier study of boys (Biederman et al., 1992), with trends toward increased alcohol abuse and drug dependence in adolescence. Although more study is needed, Biederman writes that there may be a gender-specific risk of substance abuse for girls with AD/HD—that is, that adolescent girls with AD/HD may be even more susceptible than boys with AD/HD to developing a substance use disorder. Of additional concern, Biederman and colleagues report that girls with AD/HD have a four times greater risk of smoking in adolescence, compared to teenage girls without AD/HD.

Such worrisome reports will, one hopes, motivate more parents, teachers and other professionals to work toward a better diagnostic procedure that can identify girls with AD/HD in order that they can be diagnosed, treated, and thereby avoid some of these most damaging patterns associated with AD/HD in girls.

Self-blame and shame

Just as mothers are more critical of AD/HD behaviors in their daughters, girls with AD/HD tend to internalize this criticism, leading to a strong sense of shame and self-blame. Research suggests that women, after they have progressed beyond their impulse-driven adolescent years, are much more likely than men to feel a sense of shame or humiliation as they look back on their earlier impulsive behaviors (Johnson et al., 1986). This shame seems driven by two factors: first, by the tendency of women with depression to engage in self-blame; and second, by the double standard of the society in which they live. Many in our society react with humor, even admiration to impulsive exploits on the part of males, while condemning similar behavior in females. Recent research supports this observed difference, finding that women with AD/HD struggle much more with a negative self-image than do men with AD/HD (Arcia & Conners, 1998). Typically, it is this ingrained low self-regard and lack of faith in one's acceptability that results in the greatest long-term damage from AD/HD. With good self-esteem, the challenge of learning to manage problematic AD/HD traits can be greatly reduced.

Sexual risks

Many girls with AD/HD, either through impulsivity, efforts to seek acceptance, or both, tend to engage in sexual activity earlier than their peers without AD/HD. And teenage girls with AD/HD who are emotionally volatile, impulsive, and often hungry for peer acceptance are much less likely to weigh the potentially tragic consequences of sex without birth control than are their non-AD/HD counterparts. As a result, girls with AD/HD are at much greater risk for teen pregnancy than are girls without AD/HD (Arnold, 1996).

Because girls with AD/HD run the risk of pregnancy, they potentially face much greater challenges than boys as they enter the uncharted territory of adolescent sexuality. Realistic planning and foresight are rarely among the strengths of adolescent girls with AD/HD. Yet many of them will be forced to choose among difficult decisions—to abort a pregnancy, to maintain a pregnancy, giving the child up for adoption, or to take on the responsibilities of motherhood, for which they are even less prepared than their non-AD/HD counterparts. Better treatment programs for adolescent girls with AD/HD, discussed at greater length in Chapter Ten, could help reduce the risk of teen pregnancy.

Differing parental responses

Less concerned

Even with increased awareness of girls with AD/HD, boys are more likely to be identified and to receive treatment earlier. One study shows that in girls and boys with equal degrees of inattentiveness, parents of the boys were more likely to seek treatment for their children than were parents of inattentive girls (McGee et al., 1987). The reasons for this are unclear, but one possibility is that parents and teachers alike continue to give a higher priority to the behavioral and academic functioning of boys.

Less accepting

When Russell Barkley studied parental responses to children with AD/HD, he found that mothers tend to be more critical of their daughters with AD/HD, than of their sons (Barkley, 1991). Mothers seem to find that AD/HD behaviors are more acceptable in boys, perhaps because they are more consistent with male sex role stereotypes. Girls who are messy, argumentative, explosive, or disorganized are less accepted. This finding has significant implications because patterns of frequent parental criticism and chronic rejection can result in lifelong low self-esteem and under-functioning.

Hormonal influences

Hormonal changes occurring at puberty affect emotional volatility, leading many girls with AD/HD to become emotionally hyper-reactive. Huessy (1990) writes that behavioral problems for many girls with AD/HD only begin after puberty, accompanied by an increase in emotional over-reactivity, mood swings, and impulsivity. This is a critical finding. Girls, whose behavioral problems only begin after puberty, calls into question the DSM-IV diagnostic requirement that evidence of AD/HD problems must exist prior to age seven in order to receive an AD/HD diagnosis.

The rates of anxiety and depression in AD/HD girls increase as they pass through late adolescence. This pattern of increased symptomatology in adolescence is in contrast to boys, whose hyperactivity is likely to reduce as they pass through puberty into adolescence. This pattern is of critical importance, and helps explain the later diagnosis of AD/HD in some girls.

Conclusion

Our definition and understanding of Attention Deficit/Hyperactivity Disorder has undergone many changes over the years, leading to modified nomenclature and diagnostic criteria. These changes have arisen from the scientific process of making clinical observations and from re-thinking the disorder based on those observations. In this book, we are offering our observations of girls with AD/HD and the recollections of women with AD/HD to serve as a starting point for re-thinking the diagnostic criteria as they stand today. All of these observations deserve careful study, but we cannot wait for definitive answers before we begin to address the needs of girls with AD/HD. Let us begin where we are, with careful clinical observation, and work together, as clinicians, educators, physicians, and parents to help these girls become the best they can be.

Chapter Three

Brain Development and Biologic Factors

The Brain and AD/HD

The brain is a marvelous organ. We are just beginning to understand some of its powers and functions, yet much remains a mystery. It is the place of origin for all our thoughts, behaviors, dreams, and desires, and the seat of memory and learning. Symptoms and behaviors recognized as characteristic of AD/HD are brain-based, as well, and most likely the result of differences found in specific areas of the brain. In order to understand the nature of a girl with AD/HD, it is imperative that we take a look at her brain, its formation, and subsequent development, including any gender differences and hormonal effects.

Brain development

Cell growth and death

The billions of cells (neurons) in the mature brain arise from a single layer of cells that come from the ectoderm (outer cell layer) of the embryo during the third and fourth weeks after conception, a time when most women don't even know that they are pregnant. These cells continue to multiply and the rate of increase peaks around 14 weeks after conception. Somewhere around the sixth month of pregnancy, the brain of the fetus contains the same number of cells as the adult brain. These cells continue to multiply, and an overproduction results by the time of birth. An exception to this prenatal development occurs in the cells of the cerebellum, a separate area at the base of the brain, which continue to multiply until the infant is about 10 to 11 months old.

In understanding brain development one must also understand cell death. In many other areas of the body (probably to insure its survival), there is an overproduction of cells. This overproduction occurs during brain development as well. As a rule, these surplus brain cells seem to die at the time that they establish their connections with other cells. It is this cell death (pruning) that seems to give areas of the brain their specificity. In the brain, a small, neatly packed arrangement of interconnecting cells makes for efficient transmissions and usually assures that a certain area will perform a specific function.

Brain growth and development

During the early phase of brain development, the cells (neurons) migrate to specific areas and form into groups within these areas. Linking takes place between these neurons and other areas throughout the brain by the formation of a rich network of fibers that connect individual cells and make up the various interconnecting pathways. There is also a bridge of fibers called the corpus callosum that connects the two sides (hemispheres) of the brain. The functioning of the brain depends on the connection of circuits consisting of networks of neurons. Transmission from one neuron to the next occurs at a specialized point called a synapse. Chemicals (neurotransmitters) are secreted by one neuron, cross the synapse, and are taken up by and excite the 'connected' neuron. Each neuron may be acted upon by as many as 1,000 other neurons. A single neuron may have as many as 1,000 to 10,000 points of contact with other cells. This rich network is necessary to transmit the signals and to carry on the work of the brain.

Prenatal and early brain development

Although all of the neurons of the brain are present at birth, the brain continues to grow. Cells migrate, new interconnections are made, and pruning (cell death) takes place long after birth. This process may even continue over the entire life span. However, the most rapid and vulnerable period of brain growth is from birth to approximately four years of age. That is the time when the brain is most susceptible to injury from infections and from environmental toxins such as lead.

It is now known that almost half of all premature and low birth weight infants experience later learning disabilities and AD/HD. These findings cannot be explained by social class or poor parenting, but are most likely the result of the lack of opportunity for cell production in the womb, combined with the many complex medical difficulties the baby encounters after birth. These include inadequate nutrition, infections, and injury to the brain from bleeding and/or lack of oxygen. Although the brain continues to grow after the age of four, by the age of ten or eleven, the brain has reached 95% of its adult size.

Evidence for a neurobiologic basis for AD/HD

Development of new techniques to study the brain

While no single area of the brain has been found to account for all of the symptoms of AD/HD, interconnections or neuron pathways that involve the neurotransmitter dopamine have been implicated in the behaviors seen in individuals with AD/HD for many years. Recently, neuroscientists have developed techniques that can indirectly look at the brain without damaging it. These new techniques allow us to look at what areas of the brain are turned on or off as a person performs tasks, or to take a picture to measure the size of various areas of the brain. We can even determine how much blood is flowing to various areas of the brain when a person is either at rest or engaged in a task. Almost everyone is familiar by now with the famous work of Dr. Zametkin and his coworkers at NIH (Zametkin, 1990). Using one of these new techniques, they were able to demonstrate that the brains of adults with AD/HD were not working at the same rate as those without AD/HD.

Research studies on boys

While most of the research we have today has involved only boys with AD/HD, nevertheless, it remains valuable in understanding what is going on in the brain of a person with AD/HD. Specific differences related to girls will be presented later in this chapter, but more research needs to be done on this population. The majority of research to date has shown an involvement of the frontal and prefrontal lobes of the brain (those parts of the brain behind the forehead) and the areas to which they connect in the deeper parts of the brain (sub-cortical/striatum areas). These are the areas specifically linked to motivation and emotional control—two brain functions that are adversely affected when a person has AD/HD. The executive functions of the brain, particularly attention, impulsive control, goal-orientation, and problem-solving behaviors are also known to be dependent on the prefrontal lobes and these sub-cortical connections.

Differences in brain structure

Several studies have found differences, both in these frontal areas and the corpus callosum in boys with AD/HD. Parts of the corpus callosum were found to be smaller in boys with AD/HD (Hynd et al., 1990, 1991). Disruption in the corpus callosum has long been implicated in cases of learning disabilities. It is certainly not surprising, then, that such a disruption was also found in boys with AD/HD because of the high incidence of learning disabilities that accompany AD/HD. However, these findings are important for two other reasons. First, they suggest that symptoms seen in AD/HD may be the result of differences in brain structures, and second, these variations most likely reflect problems of formation or interconnection arising during brain development. Regardless of the cause, these structural differences are most likely permanent, and are the reason that most of the symptoms of AD/HD last throughout life.

Another series of studies compared the brains of boys with

AD/HD to those without AD/HD (Filipek et al., 1997; Castellanos et al., 1996). These studies have found similar results with only minor variations. Boys with AD/HD had slightly smaller brains overall and decreased in size (volume) of certain areas of the brain known to be part of the dopamine pathways. What can we conclude from these studies? The differences found in the size of various brain structures suggest to us that AD/HD is a permanent condition that can be linked to the periods (prenatal and infancy) when development of these structures took place. These alterations in brain structures are the direct result of influences on the brain during development, the origin of which are unknown, but while most likely are the result of genetic predisposition or insults to the brain from other sources such as prematurity, infections, exposure to lead, and so on. It is also important to note that, while all of these studies found smaller size in various structures, none of the studies found any evidence of brain damage. Further, it should be pointed out that poor parenting, occurring at a later period in the child's life, could not have caused these differences in brain structures.

Gender differences in brain structure

But what are the gender differences, if any, seen in the female versus the male brain? To answer this questions let us look at several other recent studies. One such study measured the size of various brain structures in 30 children (15 males and 15 females) ages 7 to 11 years with a mean age of 9 years (Caviness et al., 1996). This study found that the brain at this age is 95% the volume of an adult brain. As in other areas of the body, the female brain was usually slightly smaller than the male brain, but the size was proportional and not significant.

The female brain usually weighs less than the male brain for the same reason that her liver and kidneys are smaller and weigh less. Her head size is smaller, just as her foot size is smaller. This proportionally smaller size relationship held up in most areas, but there were some significant exceptions. There were certain areas where the female brain was larger than the male brain. The caudate, hippocampus, and pallidum were all disproportionately larger in the female than in the male child's brain and the amygdala was disproportionately smaller in the female brain. Differences in these structures would be expected to be one of the reasons for the differing patterns of strength and weakness seen in females versus males, and might also be the cause of the variable symptom presentations in certain disorders, including AD/HD.

Cell over-population—pruning in boys

Other differences in the male versus female brain were seen at this age. The frontal lobes were at adult cell volume in females, but greater than adult volume in males, indicating that pruning (cell death) still must take place for boys. The area of the brain that held the interconnecting fibers, on the other hand, was smaller than adult levels in young females, indicating that growth in this area must be greater in females than males to reach adult volumes. These findings confirm earlier studies that also demonstrated that the brains of boys have a greater overproduction of cells that shrink as a result of pruning during adolescence in boys, but not in girls. It is this pruning that seems to assure an increase in specificity, the more efficient functioning of neuron pathways in the brain, and a decrease in symptoms clinically.

Animal studies also can give us clues as to what happens

during brain development in female versus male brains. One such study (Anderson et al., 1997) assessed the number of dopamine receptors in male and female rats from puberty into adulthood. They found that males had greater overproduction and elimination of these receptors than did females.

Differences in dopamine receptors

These gender differences in the development of the dopamine system may have significant implications regarding the gender differences seen in AD/HD. As these researchers have suggested, the overproduction of dopamine receptors during prepubertal development may help explain why males are more often afflicted with AD/HD and Tourette's syndrome than females. It is the dopamine increases in these areas that can produce hyperactivity and stereotypic motor movement or tics. Likewise, the extensive pruning that occurs during adolescence might help explain why symptoms of hyperactivity diminish in severity in males after puberty. And most importantly, the failure of receptor density to recede in females may explain why AD/HD symptoms are more likely to persist in females after puberty.

There is also emerging evidence that abnormal regulation of these patterns of brain development because of sex hormone differences can be associated with an increase in psychological and behavioral disorders. This research will be discussed further in the section on AD/HD in puberty.

Effects of estrogen on brain development

We have known for many years that estrogen affects the sex organs. It is only recently that we have discovered that estrogen also affects the brain. Both boy and girl fetuses are subjected to high levels of estrogen while in the uterus during the early phases of brain development. After birth, both males and females produce estrogen. However, females have as much as three to ten times the levels of estrogen as males. It is in girls, especially, that we must consider the effects of all of this estrogen on brain maturation and function. McEwen and co-workers, in 1997, reported that ovarian steroids have effects throughout the brain, including on the dopamine—and serotonin—(two of the hundreds of neurotransmitters) sensitive pathways. Estrogen has been shown to stimulate a significant increase in dopamine receptors. Fink and coworkers (1996) have demonstrated that estrogen also stimulates a significant increase in serotonin-binding sites.

Sensitivity to changes in estrogen levels

Receptors and binding sites are important because the more receptors we have, the more responsive a system will be to even a small amount of a transmitter. If in some conditions, such as AD/HD or depression, the amount of the transmitter is low, having more receptors or enhancing the sensitivity (turning up the volume) of these receptors would lead to a decrease in symptoms. We also know that the female brain is sensitive to low estrogen conditions (e.g. premenstrual, postpartum, and menopause) during which mood swings, irritability, sleep disorders, and other cognitive problems are seen. It is these low-estrogen states that may present an added burden for girls and women with AD/HD after puberty and menopause. The decreasing levels of estrogen seen at these times may result in a "lowering of the volume" of the receptors in girls and women that are already compromised by lowered levels of transmitters (dopamine and/or serotonin) and/or by having smaller functioning brain areas (prefrontal and inter-connecting sub-cortical areas). A worsening of the symptoms of AD/HD, an increase in mood disorders, and impaired cognitive functioning may then be seen.

Huessy, in 1990, first addressed the issue of hormones and their relationship to AD/HD by noting that girls with AD/HD may have increasingly severe problems with the onset of puberty. He wrote that increased hormonal fluctuations throughout the phases of the menstrual cycle result in increased AD/HD symptomatology. In addition, more severe PMS including increased irritability and mood swings has been reported in adolescent girls with AD/HD. Rage reactions, depression, and anxiety have also been reported to worsen during the pre-menstrual period. While 20% to 30% of the general female population experiences PMS symptoms, that number seems much higher in girls and women with AD/HD.

Anecdotal reports indicate that many women with AD/HD can remain quite functional until they enter menopause, with its concomitant decrease in hormone levels, at which time, they no longer are able to cope as effectively with their AD/HD symptoms. Despite these reports, until we study girls and women with AD/HD and the effects of puberty, menopause, and varying hormone levels, we may not have the answers to many of these questions.

Increasing symptoms of AD/HD in girls at puberty

Puberty is a time of great turmoil and change. As the brain approaches maturity, it is exposed to a dramatic increase in adrenal hormones during adrenarche (awakening of the adrenal glands) and a year or two later, to an increase in sex hormones (testosterone and estadiol) during gonadarche (breast and genital development). These hormonal changes at puberty have long been blamed for the mood and behavior changes seen at this time. In studying a group of children who had premature adrenarche (turning on of the adrenal glands, but not sexual development), researchers were able to study the effect of hormones without the interference of social factors on behaviors. In this study, it was found that the children with earlier onset of the start of puberty also had significantly higher levels of all the hormones (adrenal androgens, estradiol, and cortisol) than children who began the process at the age-appropriate times. It was also reported that the children with these higher-than-normal levels of hormones had significant psychosocial problems, including anxiety/ depression, attention and behavior problems, impaired cognitive functioning, and school performance (Dorn et al., 1999). In other studies, girls with early maturation (precocious puberty) were shown to have more internalizing and externalizing behavior problems (Sonis, 1985).

AD/HD in most cases is present from birth, but for many girls the symptomatology of AD/HD does not become bothersome until they reach puberty. A worsening of symptoms of AD/HD may be seen at that time. In addition, a girl's impaired executive functioning may manifest only then as disorganization and performance worsen in response to life's increasing demands. Mothers report that their daughters experience a significant increase in irritability and mood swings starting at puberty. However, to date, no studies have been undertaken in girls with AD/HD to determine if the worsening of symptoms they exhibit may be related to higher-than-normal levels of adrenal and sex hormones during puberty.

Girls more likely to be referred for LD than AD/HD

As their cognitive dysfunction becomes more prominent in middle school, resulting in more academic difficulties, girls may be referred by their teachers for evaluation of possible learning disabilities. Such a referral appears to be a more common occurrence than a referral for AD/HD. This may be the reason that some studies of girls with AD/HD have reported that girls have a higher incidence of learning disabilities than do boys with AD/HD (Gaub & Carlson, 1997). This increased incidence, however, may be simply a referral bias resulting from the fact that it is their poor academic achievement that gets these girls referred for evaluations, not their symptoms of AD/HD—that is, if they get referred at all. Some girls may be thought of as just not as bright or academically capable as others. These experiences initiate the poor sense of self-esteem and lack of awareness of their own capabilities frequently seen in girls and women with AD/HD.

A study of younger girls with AD/HD (Seidman et al., 1997) did not find as great a degree of executive dysfunction as in boys, but this may be a factor of the ages of the girls studied. The girls may have been "too young" to manifest the symptoms of brain dysfunction to the degree often seen after the onset of puberty. An earlier study of adolescent girls (Ernst, Zametkin et al., 1994) has found that brain dysfunction measured by glucose metabolism was correlated with Tanner stage (the degree to which a girl had entered puberty as measured by breast and pubic hair changes). The further along the development of these secondary sexual characteristics, the greater was the brain dysfunction, regardless of the girl's chronological age. This study has not been replicated, but it seems to deal with similar issues as those studies presented earlier about the correlation and timing of psychological and behavior disturbances in girls with higher than normal levels of hormones during puberty.

Delayed symptoms in girls calls DSM-IV criteria into question

The delayed presentation of symptoms and cognitive impairments until puberty in many girls with AD/HD demands that we call into question the DSM-IV criteria that the onset of symptoms must take place before age seven in order for the diagnosis of AD/HD to be made. Joseph Beiderman and Russell Barkley have recently recommended that the threshold for onset be raised to at least thirteen years—and that even that be loosely adhered to—in keeping with the concept that the onset occurs during childhood, but can occur beyond age seven (Barkley, 1997). This concept may prove especially true for girls with the disorder.

Improving the identification of girls

Over the years, girls with AD/HD have been overlooked because experts were focusing on the classic symptoms of hyperactivity and impulsivity. With the advent of DSM-IV and the preceding field trials, it became apparent that AD/HD, without these classic symptoms of hyperactivity and impulsivity, does exist and that more girls are found in that subgroup. In these trials, girls made up 20% of the hyperactive/impulsive group, 27% of the inattentive group, and 12% of the combined type group (Lahey & Carlson, 1991). Even in this study, we are probably under-representing the numbers of girls with AD/HD

In reviewing the studies to date that focus on the inattentive type, Barkley suggests that the inattentive subtype may have more problems with the focused or selective component of attention. They may appear sluggish and less accurate in information processing and have memory retrieval problems. In addition, they may have more anxiety and mood disorders, and are often rated as shy, withdrawn, reticent, or apprehensive. He reiterates that it remains unclear to whether differences exist in sex ratios in the various subtypes of AD/HD, though males seem to predominate (Barkley, 1997). However, Barkley's description certainly fits many of the girls we see with AD/HD.

Conclusion

AD/HD is a neurologically based condition. As such, it is directly affected by influences on the brain during critical developmental periods. During these times, the brain is most susceptible to injury and other insults. For example, premature and low birth weight infants frequently experience later learning disabilities and AD/HD. These findings cannot be explained by social class or poor parenting, but are most likely the result of the insults to the infant in the womb combined with the many complex medical difficulties the baby encounters after birth.

Differences in the male versus female brain exist and have been documented in animal studies and in research conducted on elementary school aged children. More importantly, as the brain approaches maturity, it is exposed to significant hormonal bombardment from both the adrenals and sex organs. Do gender differences in the development of the dopamine and serotonin receptor systems result? What other factors contribute to significant gender differences seen in AD/HD?

To date, few studies have been conducted to assess such important factors and their implications. It, therefore, becomes imperative that parents, teachers, physicians, and mental health professionals join together and raise their voices to call on researchers to address these issues if we are ever to truly understand AD/HD in girls.

Chapter Four

AD/HD in Girls: Far More Than Meets the Eye

As described in previous chapters, the majority of children diagnosed with AD/HD are boys. Data from predominantly male AD/HD clinic populations has formed the bases for most studies. Research results often are reported by the media without reference to gender, sending the implicit message that the results pertain just as equally to girls as to boys. But do they? Gender research highlighting the differences between the experiences of girls and boys should lead us to question the validity of this assumption and to be concerned about its impact.

While there is an abundance of information available on AD/HD, we know less about the experience of girls with AD/HD than we may assume that we do. While AD/HD was first described in 1902 in the British journal, *The Lancet* (Still,

1902), it was not until 1980 that the name of the disorder came to reflect the possibility of AD/HD without hyperactivity. It is not surprising, then, that prior to 1980, a negligible number of girls were diagnosed with attentional problems.

Since 1980, each edition of the Diagnostic and Statistical Manual has revised the conceptualization of AD/HD to reflect the current thinking (American Psychiatric Association, 1968, 1980, 1987, 1994). In the DSM-IV (American Psychiatric Association, 1994), AD/HD is grouped with the Disruptive Behavior Disorders, a strong reflection of the current emphasis on the more typically male presentation of the disorder. The DSM-IV identifies three subtypes, based on the predominant features expressed. While the different subtypes will be addressed under these headings for convention, note that we do not conceptualize them as hard and fast categories. Most girls with AD/HD will probably be some composite of the descriptions. Additionally, as we will highlight throughout this book, there are a range of emotional and cognitive patterns in girls with AD/HD that are not addressed within the current DSM-IV framework.

Predominantly hyperactive-impulsive type

It is easiest to spot the hyperactive girls whose symptoms are similar to those of many boys with AD/HD. They compose only a small percentage of girls with AD/HD, although they are probably the majority of girls that are brought to clinics for evaluation. They are the loud, physically active, intrusive and demanding risk takers. Many are defiant, aggressive and often invade the personal space of their peers. They may be found in the emergency room getting stitches or being treated for a concussion much more frequently that their non-AD/HD peers. They may be the girls in class who are told by an exasperated teacher to stay in their seat and stop turning around. Because their behaviors are in stark contrast to the quiet and compliant stereotype of a "typical" girl, such girls will be very visible to teachers and parents.

Many girls with the hyperactive/ impulsive subtype of AD/ HD are described by their parents as being 'different' or 'difficult' by the age of three or four years. Their hyperactive behaviors that may first attract attention are often a disappointment to parents. While wild behavior is expected in young boys, parents often feel embarrassed by girls who engage in similar behaviors. Studies show that there is generally harsher criticism of girls with these behaviors than of boys (Barkley et al.,1992). These girls may find social success by being an aggressive player on the soccer or basketball team. While this can make them sought after as a star athlete, temper tantrums also may be a part of this intense symptom picture. For some girls a pattern of tantrums, willfulness and emotional intensity places them in a subgroup that may require different treatment interventions, both in terms of medication and non-medication treatment.

They may have a higher percentage of learning problems than the other subtypes of girls with AD/HD (Seidman et al., 1997). Their rooms and their school desks are messy and often their handwriting is poor. They may write over margins, run words together without spaces, or forget to skip lines between items. Sometimes the fine motor control necessary to write with a pencil is uncomfortable for them, and they may find it difficult to control the size of letters and the pressure on the paper. These are the children who shake out the kinks in their hands after every few lines they write. Indeed, their homework is a reflection of the chaotic way that information is stored in their minds. The answers may be right, but it is the intrepid teacher who will sift through and decode a paper that may appear to be dashed off by a girl who doesn't care.

Combined type

Many girls with AD/HD conform more to gender role expectations, and behave in ways that are less aggressive, less defiant, and less rebellious than are boys. This more frequent presentation of girls with AD/HD includes those who appear restless, fidgety, and "hyperreactive" rather than overtly hyperactive. At school, they may be extremely talkative and giggly; a report card comment may read "has trouble working quietly." A teacher's suggestion might read, "if she would buckle down and try harder, she could work up to her potential." They may be excitable, interrupt others frequently, jump from topic to topic without obvious segues, or persevere endlessly on a given topic. Because they are so dramatic and controlling, they may be viewed by their peers as charismatic social leaders, or, alternatively, as bossy, stubborn, and spoiled.

They may be emotionally over reactive with mood swings, intense arguments, or tears. Once upset, their anger can escalate like a flash-fire, and they may resort to ultimatums like, "I don't ever want to talk to you again" and "You're the meanest person I've ever met." At home they may be irritable, moody and unmotivated, with a low frustration tolerance. Some girls may experience extraordinary difficulty in getting up and out of the house, resulting in repeated school tardiness. They may make it clear that they are completely unsatisfied with their life, and it may be "all your fault." Another common coping style is to adopt a "silly" persona with peers, to mask their disorganization, forgetfulness, and confusion. Those not confident enough to be either a social leader or a bully, may adopt a submissive role that at least succeeds in maintaining relationships, rather than alienating others.

Predominantly inattentive type

Perhaps the majority of girls with AD/HD fall into the primarily inattentive type, and are most likely to go undiagnosed. Generally, these girls are more compliant than disruptive and get by rather passively in the academic arena. They may be hypoactive or lethargic. In the extreme, they may even seem narcoleptic. Because they do not appear to stray from cultural norms, they will rarely come to the attention of their teacher.

Early report cards of an inattentive type girl may read, "She is such a sweet little girl. She must try harder to speak up in class." She is often a shy daydreamer who avoids drawing attention to herself. Fearful of expressing herself in class, she is concerned that she will be ridiculed or wrong. She often feels awkward, and may nervously twirl the ends of her hair. Her preferred seating position is in the rear of the classroom. She may appear to be listening to the teacher, even when she has drifted off and her thoughts are far away. These girls avoid challenges, are easily discouraged, and tend to give up quickly. Their lack of confidence in themselves is reflected in their failure excuses, such as, "I can't," "It's too hard," or "I used to know it, but I can't remember it now."

The inattentive girl is likely to be disorganized, forgetful, and often anxious about her school work. Teachers may be frustrated because she does not finish class work on time. She may mistakenly be judged as less bright than she really is. These girls are reluctant to volunteer for a project or join a group of peers at recess. They worry that other children will humiliate them if they make a mistake, which they are sure they will. Indeed, one of their greatest fears is being called on in class; they may stare down at their book to avoid eye contact with the teacher, hoping that the teacher will forget they exist for the moment.

Because interactions with the teacher are often anxiety-ridden, these girls may have trouble expressing themselves, even when they know the answer. Sometimes, it is concluded that they have problems with central auditory processing or expressive language skills. More likely, their anxiety interferes with their concentration, temporarily reducing their capacity to both speak and listen. Generally, these girls don't experience this problem around family or close friends, where they are more relaxed.

Inattentive type girls with a high IQ and no learning disabilities will be diagnosed with AD/HD very late, if ever. These bright girls have the ability and the resources to compensate for their cognitive challenges, but it's a mixed blessing. Their psychological distress is internalized, making it less obvious, but no less damaging. Some of these girls will go unnoticed until college or beyond, and many are never diagnosed—they are left to live with chronic stress that may develop into anxiety and depression as their exhausting, hidden efforts to succeed take their toll.

Issues for girls with AD/HD

In the remainder of this chapter, we will present a range of issues for girls with AD/HD that are relevant, regardless of developmental stage. In the chapters that follow, we will focus on patterns and issues of particular relevance at each succeeding developmental stage, from toddler-hood through high school.

Lags in maturation

At every point in their development, girls with AD/HD are challenged to make "age-appropriate" transitions at a so-cially-accepted pace. With each new developmental stage, there are skills to master. However, these new skills do not come easily to the girl with AD/HD; in fact, some of the requisite skills develop at a torturously slow pace, with significant repercussions at home, at school, and with peers.

There are many lags in skill development with which AD/HD girls must cope. In combination, these lags explain why girls with AD/HD are often considered immature for their age. These lags are often manifested in their greater comfort in playing with younger children, or their contentedness with a younger sibling's toys. It may take them longer to consistently tell time on an analog clock, to reliably distinguish left from right, and to organize their backpacks for school. While they may practice these skills with the guidance of supportive adults, there may be many painful trial-and-errors first. They often ask themselves, "Why are things that seem easy for everyone else so hard for me?"

Parents can play an encouraging and supportive role by reminding their daughters that everyone learns at their own pace, reassuring them that they will develop new skills with time and practice. Often parents need such reassurance themselves, from a professional, before they can pass it along to their daughters.

Lags in maturation typically continue into adolescence and

young adulthood. Girls with AD/HD may not be ready to drive at 16; they may not be ready to leave home for college at 18; and, they may not be ready for a smooth transition to independent living as early as a girl without AD/HD. The parent who is comfortably aware of this developmental difference is better able to reassure her daughter, when she is frustrated in trying to "keep up with" peers, and to appropriately support her as she develops the skills necessary for independent living.

Applying learning to new situations

Many girls with AD/HD have difficulty applying skills or strategies that they have learned in one situation to a similar situation. For example, Fran has gradually learned how important it is for her to get enough sleep on school nights in order to function well the next day. However, when Fran spends Friday night with Amy before an important soccer match on Saturday morning, this knowledge may not be applied. It's not a "school night" so Fran stays up late and is in no shape to play her best the next day. Rather than grumbling, "You should have known better," when Fran's mom picks up a tired daughter on Saturday morning, Fran needs concrete reminders, regardless of how smart she may be. "If you're going to spend the night with Amy, you have to promise to be in bed by eleven, no matter what."

Because every new situation poses a new problem to be solved, it is very challenging for a girl with AD/HD to create a more predictable world for herself. An attuned adult may need to serve as the bridge between relevant experiences in order to help her generalize her experience to other situations. "Remember how tired you were last time you stayed up? Remember that the coach was annoyed with you for not paying attention during the game?"

Self-monitoring

Another critical skill needed as a building block for appropriate behavior is the ability to self-monitor—to observe one's own behavior, evaluate its appropriateness in relation to others, and adjust it, as needed, in a given situation. This skill is one of the most difficult for girls with AD/HD to master consistently, and it requires a tremendous amount of practice. It is also a skill that most people assume is in place when it's not.

For example, a girl with AD/HD may be perceptive about others, and self-observant in certain situations, but unable to monitor her behavior in other situations. Fielding novel stimuli can be overwhelming and confusing for the girl with AD/HD; so much energy is devoted to reacting that the task of self-observation is forced to take a backseat.

Parents, teachers, and professionals can help girls become more self-aware through rehearsal and "instant replay." One interesting therapeutic technique, discussed in a later chapter, uses a video camera to help girls with AD/HD identify their impact in interactions with others.

Managing simultaneous events

Another AD/HD detour on the road to smooth cognitive development is having difficulty keeping track of more than one thing at a time. Because all stimuli are equally compelling, one of the hardest tasks for a girl with AD/HD is to set priorities. Whatever her current focus (e.g., the squirrel outside the classroom window), it is usually to the exclusion of competing stimuli (e.g., the teacher describing the homework assignment). With a rich kaleidoscope of stimuli swirling around her, prioritizing is a challenging task.

Indeed, it is difficult to filter out the extraneous stimuli and select the one that is most important. This is a loaded decision because the object of focus deemed most important by society is not necessarily the one that is inherently most interesting to the girl with AD/HD. Because the "correct" stimuli may not stimulate her brain enough, she does not feel motivated to pay attention to it. The cognitive struggle, then, is not about distractibility or a short attention span; it is a struggle to regulate attention, and to selectively screen out stimuli that may have great inherent interest and maintain attention to a less interesting stimuli.

Parents and others can help girls with AD/HD become aware of their difficulty in juggling more than one thing at a time. The TV may need to be turned off while a toddler or young child picks up toys. Similarly, a teenage girl with AD/HD may need to practice her driving skills for a long period of time, without the distraction of other teens in the car, before she can safely talk and drive at the same time.

Managing transitions

Transitions are notoriously difficult for all children with AD/HD. After finally adjusting to the structure of the school day, a girl with AD/HD is then faced with the chaotic bus ride home, and the structure-less "downtime" of home. After holding herself together during the whole school day, there is a physical, mental, and emotional release when she reaches the safe haven of home. Generally, she will do best with a period of time to "chill." Some girls are 'starving' for a snack (especially true if she is taking a stimulant that wears off at the end of the school day). This decompression time is critical to allow her, without further demands, to establish a new equilibrium at home.

Parents are often fearful that if homework is not begun soon after arrival home from school that it will never be completed. Despite this risk, girls with AD/HD need decompression time. A younger girl may need to actively play outside, or relax in front of the TV. Teens with AD/HD, often chronically sleep deprived, may even need a nap before they can focus on homework.

The importance of structure

Many AD/HD children are too overwhelmed at the end of a school day to deal with an unstructured and demanding interaction with a friend. Creating an after-school routine is very helpful for girls with AD/HD. For example, unstructured downtime should be of a predictable length, and she must know that homework follows the circumscribed period of downtime. Similarly, if dinner is always at 7:00, there is less likelihood of, "it's too early," "I need five more minutes," or "I'm not hungry yet."

Without a built-in motivator, few girls with AD/HD will overcome their inertia and change gears to start a new activity. In fact, especially if she is at the rigid end of the continuum, there may be significant resistance to transitions.

Low-key and friendly statements like, "in 15 minutes it's going to be time to turn off the computer and go upstairs to take a shower" can help avert an unpleasant power struggle between parent and child. These advance notices from an attuned parent also can prevent her from feeling ambushed and out of control at home. Teachers often announce routine transitions by turning the lights on and off or playing a brief musical phrase. These communications actually empower the AD/HD girl who feels proud that she knows exactly what is transpiring and is not in a state of confusion. Similarly, at home, the more information you can give a girl with AD/HD about what to expect, what constitutes acceptable behavior, and what the consequences are for unacceptable behavior, the safer and more predictable her world will feel to her.

The importance of modulating stimulation levels

This struggle to find the "right" level of stimulation is ongoing in a girl with AD/HD. At one pole, she craves high stimulation for her senses. Her brain reaches its highest level of alertness when she confronts novelty. In other words, she is neurologically driven to push the limits of the envelope for the thrill it provides. Under-stimulation, or "boredom" is a state in which her brain is not aroused for optimum functioning. In fact, in an under-stimulating, mundane situation, she may create noise, color, excitement, chaos, or conflict if there is no other stimulation available.

Unable to carefully modulate the level of stimulation she needs for optimal functioning, she tends to go too far to a state of over-stimulation, which may lead to tears or disaster before she seeks the comfort of a less stimulating environment. Suddenly, the fun becomes too much fun, the laughter takes on a hint of hysteria, sights and sounds bombard her until she feels disoriented. Now she panics, and desperately needs to withdraw to a place where there are no demands placed on her, no interaction expected, and no extraneous stimuli. In essence, she is craving the opportunity to shut down and regroup her forces. The pendulum careens back in the other direction. After stirring up commotion, suddenly she wants everyone to leave her alone.

Sometimes disaster can be averted if the observant parent or teacher calms the situation before it reaches "overload" proportions by anticipating the triggers that a child finds over-whelming and helping her circumvent them. Girls with AD/HD, and even women with AD/HD, left to their own de-vices, may not see the "crash" coming until they are emo-tionally or physically exhausted.

This description illustrates the inconsistent sensory per-ceptions of her world that provoke so many to be dubious of the phenomenon of AD/HD. How can she be so consistently inconsistent? As is always the case with a girl with AD/HD, sometimes she responds too much, and sometimes not enough; this immense struggle to monitor and regulate her responses is the very hallmark of AD/HD.

The impact of a hyper-sensitive central nervous system

While not all girls fall into this category, the successful man-agement of a hyper-sensitive central nervous system is the primary neurobiological challenge for many girls with AD/HD.

Tactile sensitivity

Do you know a girl who will wear only leggings? Who rips the labels out of the back of her t-shirts? Who cries dra-matically following an injury that seems minimal to you? Who shrinks from being hugged? All of these can be manifesta-tions of an ultra-sensitive sense of touch, which is sometimes termed "tactile defensiveness." Clothes with tight waists, that are constricting, that are made of wool or other rough textures, are annoying to some girls with AD/HD, although they may not be fully aware of the tactile irritation. This subtle low level stimulation to the central nervous system is persistent and irritating. Some girls with AD/HD find being touched intrusive; being crowded and jostled on line to the cafeteria is almost unbearable. These may be girls who will hang back on the fringes of a group activity, and who will turn their heads away when an aunt goes to kiss them. It is not out of rudeness or aloofness, but out of a physiological need to avoid that kind of sensory over-stimulation.

Parents should take her need for comfortable clothing seriously. If she is not distracted by an irritating clothing label or the waistband of her jeans, she'll be better able to focus on her schoolwork. Respect her level of tolerance and don't insist on giving her a big hug when you arrive home each day. It may help to let her make the first move so that she is better prepared for physical contact. Also, acknowledge the many non-physical ways of expressing affection and brainstorm alternate behaviors together.

The same girl who is distracted by irritating sensations may become hyper-focused on pleasurable ones. For example, she may revel in the sensation of sitting in a tub of warm water, to the exclusion of other practical demands. After a half hour, you may find her still sitting in the tub, still unwashed, watching her feet make ripples in the water. You can help her stay on task by agreeing to a time limit beforehand, and giving a warning, such as, "You have ten more minutes; it's time to wash your hair." In general, helping her recognize the sensations she is sensitive to will help her plan coping strategies.

Physical complaints

Because these girls are so sensitive and not always in touch with their emotional status, feelings like anxiety or anger may be experienced viscerally, as somatic complaints, such as stomachaches or headaches. They may experience these or other physical symptoms far more often than same-age siblings, and parents may become concerned. As parents and doctors search for physical explanations for their discomfort, the girl's sense that she is different and incomprehensible may be reinforced. As for the screams, tears, or repetitive complaints following an injury, it is true that the same injury would probably affect others to a lesser degree. While this behavior may appear overly dramatic, it is important to remember that their senses are heightened and her discomfort is real. It is best neither to encourage this behavior nor to invalidate her experience, but to acknowledge her discomfort and treat it, if necessary.

Problems with bladder control

A tendency to urinate frequently and/or wet the bed (enuresis) can also be a manifestation of this heightened sensitivity (Biederman et al., 1995a). At one end of the continuum, a girl may sense pressure on her bladder from only a few drops of accumulated urine; nonetheless, that acute sensation may be a primary distraction until she has voided. At the other end of the continuum, many girls will wait until the last moment to relieve themselves. They are reluctant to acknowledge the pressure on their bladders until it is an "emergency" because they are hyper-focused on the activity in which they are involved. Reminders to take bathroom breaks and to "go" before getting into the car can help avert some of these crises.

Bed-wetting may be a problem, even into the early teen

years. In a common AD/HD scenario, a girl may be so deeply involved in her dream that she won't acknowledge the competing signal from her bladder. Much as she ignores you when her favorite TV show is on, she may ignore the less-interesting message and delay urination until it is too late. It is always prudent to have a thorough physical examination to rule out any physical causes for the bed-wetting. It is also useful to know that bed-wetting can increase a girl's risk of getting repeated urinary tract infections.

Above all, it is essential not to punish the child for her bed-wetting, and to let her know that she has not been bad For the fragile self-esteem of a girl with AD/HD, bed-wetting is a harsh addition to the perceived failures she is already struggling to hide. Waking a child to void her bladder before the parents go to bed may be helpful. Intake of liquids should be limited within an hour or two of bedtime. Reassure her that she'll outgrow it. It can help to tell family stories about those who wet their beds as children. "You see, Aunt Barbara doesn't wet the bed anymore, does she?"

Tastes and smells

Taste, texture, and smell sensitivities are problematic in many AD/HD households; almost universally, the food domain provides some of the most frustrating challenges. There maybe a limited number of foods that a girl with AD/HD is willing to eat. And those foods are acceptable only if they are prepared exactly as the parent prepares it. Then, there are the regulatory demands: it must be neither too hot nor too cold, nor too spicy, nor too rough a texture, nor too strong an odor, nor touching another food on the plate.

Foods bland in taste and texture are usually the most acceptable: many AD/HD girls are willing to eat macaroni and cheese (usually restricted to a single brand), soup, (especially alphabet soup, which provides another source of interest while eating), Cheerios, or a bagel.

Eating behaviors can be an area of tremendous conflict in homes with a daughter who has AD/HD. Eating is inherently an impulse-driven activity; and, with AD/HD, it is much more difficult to regulate. Like many other developmental skills, a girl with AD/HD may exhibit behaviors usually displayed by younger children. She may eat food so quickly that she'll get air in her stomach, resulting in loud belching or gas pains. If her beverage is poured first, she may finish the drink in one long gulp before the meal even begins. She may favor eating with her hands, and show little awareness of the napkin next to her plate. She may have food on her face, or a milk moustache and be unaware of it. She may ask for seconds when she hasn't even finished what's on her plate.

At the other end of the spectrum is the very picky eater. She is easily overwhelmed by the tastes, textures, and smells of foods. She may be absorbed in an activity and have little interest in stopping to eat. In fact, when she is involved in an activity, she may just forget to eat. Then, when she must shift to a boring endeavor—homework, for example—she will suddenly become aware of her hunger. This is not manipulation (for the most part). She may eat very slowly, and get more involved in playing with her food than eating it. She may say she's full, with an eye towards leaving the table as soon as possible.

Children outgrow most or all of their "picky-ness" with time. Food battles are rarely productive. A parent will do better to minimize the junk food available in the house, making a variety of healthier foods available and allowing her child to choose her diet, within reason.

Response to sound

Girls with AD/HD can appear "deaf" at times, while being exquisitely sensitive to sounds at other times. One mother said, "Sometimes I swear she's deaf because she doesn't even look up when I've said the same thing five times." This phenomenon has nothing to do with her hearing. She is simply hyper-focused on something else. Her parent's voice, with its likely message of a directive, hasn't succeeded yet in capturing her attention.

Yet, the same girl may have sensitivities to sound that create apparent eccentricities. For example, sudden loud noises may be experienced as alarming and unsettling. In addition, it takes longer for her to calm down again than it does a child without AD/HD. Many girls complain when the volume of the TV increases during a commercial. Offensive, low level annoyances include buzzing light fixtures, ticking clocks, and static on the radio. She may be more comfortable with a digital clock on her headboard. Crowded, noisy events, such as the fireworks on July 4th, may be unpleasant for her. Multiple competing sounds can be frustrating to the point of being overwhelming. The shouts, swings squeaking, and sounds of balls hitting the backboard at recess can make her irritable; she may separate herself from the fray for some relative silence in which to regroup her forces.

Yet, the same child may dance about at home, singing at the top of her lungs, or turning up the sound on her favorite TV show to a deafening level. And never underestimate, that she hears every word of what you whisper about her in the next room. Like the other senses, each girl has an optimal level of sound stimulation that is unique to her; silence is too quiet, and chaos too noisy. The noise level also includes her thoughts, and a comfortable balance is sometimes elusive.

Unrelated to this sensitivity, it is interesting to note that recurrent ear infections are about five times more likely to occur in girls with AD/HD than in their non-AD/HD counterparts. (Adesman et al., 1990).

Bodies in motion

While some girls with AD/HD are excellent athletes, other girls with AD/HD have coordination difficulties, which render them clumsy, or more likely to trip, fall or bang into furniture. These girls are less likely to feel comfortable playing sports, and they may be teased for being a "spaz."

The less coordinated girls with AD/HD tend to do best in sports that do not cross the vertical midline of the body—that is, sports that do not require her to cross her right hand or foot across to the left side of her body, or vice-versa. She will also be likely to do best at sports that do not involve teams. The more user-friendly activities include jumping rope, bicycle riding, swimming, gymnastics, martial arts, hiking and running. Involvement in one of these activities can improve skills and provide a sense of well being. It also offers a structured way of interacting with like-minded girls. You can support your daughter's attempts to practice her skills by suggesting, "Let's take a bike ride after dinner."

Many girls with AD/HD experience "flailing injuries" because their bodies and limbs are often moving in accidental fashion. Knuckles graze the wall as they dash by, knees do not quite clear the table leg, and leaping up sometimes means a bump on the head. They often feel victimized by the walls or the furniture, and there is embarrassment, as well as the all-too familiar sense that they cannot trust their own perceptions. You can help her become more aware of her body in space, and in relation to others, via gymnastics or a modern dance class. Reassure her that many children have mishaps when they are deep in thought about something else.

Obsessional behaviors

The internal experience of a girl with AD/HD is frequently one of chaotic disorganization, a whirling barrage of thoughts and feelings emanating from within, as well as a relentless stream of unfiltered external stimuli. The rapid movement of ideas cannot be slowed down, and it is sometimes hard to seize an idea of particular interest as it is whizzes by. This sense of disorganization, sometimes manifested by a messy desk, backpack, room and/or handwriting, is extremely frustrating for her, and often exasperating to others.

Some girls with AD/HD are so uncomfortable with these chaotic feelings within them that they try to find ways to compensate. One way she can avoid that out-of-control feeling is to impose obsessive order on external things. In this way, she creates a structure that increases her sense of control, but it does so at the cost of rigidity. It is also quite time-consuming to be obsessive in one's organization, and usually results in the obsessive girl being the last to finish things in class. It reduces spontaneity along with chaos. In fact, she may fear spontaneity because she feels out of control. In her search for order she blocks off many paths toward creativity.

Her obsessive controls will tend to increase as she feels more anxious and overwhelmed. Although parents may praise their daughter for her "neatness," they also should be aware that extreme obsessiveness is a sign of anxiety, and perhaps an indication that their daughter needs help in reducing the stress level in her life. When obsessiveness, like checking and rechecking, counting items or washing gets in the way of daily functioning, she may need treatment for anxiety as well as for AD/HD.

Shame

For most females, an inability to conform to cultural gender role expectations evokes feelings of shame—a phenomenon that Sari Solden writes about extensively in her book, *Women with Attention Deficit Disorder* (Solden, 1995). The girls with AD/HD who are messy, whose hair is out of place, who forget to RSVP to parties—these girls know they are different, even if they don't understand why. In elementary school, their sense of self-esteem consists of the reflected appraisals of adults and the acceptance of their peers. They make desperate attempts to compensate—with obsessive efforts toward self-control, silliness, aggression, somatic complaints like stomachaches or headaches, or withdrawal. Sadly, they learn that despite their best efforts, they cannot be consistently successful. Sadly, trying their best does not always yield the rewards they seek.

Shame is central to girls' experience of AD/HD because their disappointments and frustrations are generally held inside, rather than acted out. They feel bad, but try to hide their discomfort from the world. Little girls can become hyperfocused on their mistakes and failures when they are highlighted, perhaps inadvertently, by parents, teachers, peers, and society in general. Then, shame can begin to feed upon itself, giving way to feelings of depression and/or anxiety.

Psychological distress

Often, it is the overt symptoms of anxiety or depression that may ultimately lead to a girl being referred for help. In fact, because of those presenting problems, the AD/HD diagnosis can easily be missed. When a young girl makes hopeless statements like, "I hate my life" and "I feel worthless," she may be responding to the shame and disappointment that results from living with AD/HD. In other words, it can be truly demoralizing to realize that, regardless of how bright she is, she cannot gain complete control over her feelings or behavior.

Girls have been shown to experience more internalized psychological distress than boys (Brown et al., 1989). Secondary psychological symptoms gradually arise as a result of the anxiety and/or depression that are responses to the initial AD/HD symptoms. Anxiety and depression make the already difficult challenge of coping with AD/HD symptoms a struggle filled with emotional turmoil.

Parents and others who work with girls with AD/HD can have a positive impact upon their sense of shame by helping to re-frame their difficulties as being "just like everyone else." It is critical that girls develop a sense of themselves as "OK" by helping them to find social outlets where peers are more accepting. Finding strengths and interests and encouraging girls with AD/HD to develop those strengths can also counterbalance a sense of shame over their "different-ness." AD/HD support groups for girls can also provide a safe, supportive environment in which to gain self-acceptance while developing better social skills.

Emotional neediness

The physical, mental, and emotional needs of the girl with AD/HD may seem insatiable. Her neediness may seem like a bottomless pit, and well-meaning parents often fall into the trap of attempting to fill this pit. The end result is usually a parent, close to tears, drained of physical and emotional energy, and a girl with AD/HD, who may feel rewarded by the intense interaction with her parent.

Teachers who have to manage a class of children including three or four students with AD/HD may respond differently. While initially compassionate, they may become irritated at the constant drain on their time, energy and attention. Ultimately, there may be an element of truth when the child with AD/HD perceives that the teacher "didn't call on me today" or "sent me to the principal, but I didn't do anything." The neediness of these girls, when viewed within the broader framework of all the students in a class, may be as disruptive and unwieldy as the most aggressive student.

While girls with AD/HD *are* needier than many of their peers, they need to gradually learn techniques to calm, and gratify themselves. Support for these girls should include lessons in self-reliance. She may need to do her homework in the kitchen, where her mother's presence provides automatic structure and emotional support, but she doesn't need her mother to help her do each math problem. She may need to talk about the emotional bumps and bruises of her day, but parents will do well to help her improve her social skills during those "heart to heart" talks, rather than serve simply as a fountain of empathy. "I've got a problem," should be followed quickly by "and this is what I'll try to do about it."

Oral behaviors

Some girls with AD/HD engage in compulsive oral behaviors both as a response to their emotional neediness and as a form of fidgeting, a small-motor, less noticeable manifestation of hyperactivity. Although no formal studies have addressed the problematic eating patterns of girls with AD/HD, women with AD/HD report that eating as a self-calming or self-comforting activity is one of the most prevalent problematic eating pattern (Nadeau, 1998; Richardson, 1997; Wilens et al., 1996). While this is a developmentally-appropriate coping strategy for infants and young toddlers, it sometimes continues in girls with AD/HD, even into adulthood. Variants of oral behavior include age-inappropriate sucking or chewing on clothing, especially sleeves, buttons, necklines, or the strings from a sweatshirt hood, sucking their thumb, or biting and spitting. Or, they may tend to have something inedible in their mouths to manipulate with their tongues; frequent examples of this include biting nails and/or cuticles, sucking or chewing on the ends of their hair, or chewing on pencils or pen caps. More socially-acceptable behaviors that still satisfy oral needs include gum chewing, or sucking on mints, hard candies, or ice cubes. Later, smoking and drinking can serve this purpose. Compulsive overeating, which can begin in childhood, is yet another behavior that is meant to quell the search for oral gratification. In essence, all of these behaviors are attempts at self-soothing; in fact, these behaviors allow the girl to 'self-medicate' as a means of easing feelings of restlessness, social awkwardness, anxiety and shame.

Parents should avoid responding with harsh criticism to

behaviors such as compulsive nail-biting, but rather should view them as signs of insecurity and even of hyperactivity. Some girls need to be "doing something all the time," and will nail bite or engage in other small motor activities when they are required to sit still as they listen to the teacher or do homework. Parents can help their daughter find the least destructive way to fidget—nerf balls or other squeezable objects are often appealing. If she *wants* to stop nail biting, help her by giving her a substitute—softer, plastic ball point pen covers won't harm teeth and may help her transition away from nail-biting. As she goes into middle school and is more conscious of personal grooming, she may respond to an incentive to have a professional manicure with special nail polish if she is able to grow her nails to the desired length.

Sleep disturbance

Since fluctuating levels of arousal are a central issue, it is not surprising that girls with AD/HD may have all manner of sleep disturbances, including difficulty falling asleep, difficulty staying asleep, difficulty in awakening, and difficulty maintaining daytime alertness. Bedtime and awaking battles are among the most painful family struggles. Most girls with AD/HD resist bedtime because, although they may be physically exhausted, their minds remain overactive, and their thoughts are not slowing down in tandem with their bodies. Occasionally, stimulant medications can exacerbate a vulnerable sleep situation. In general, it takes a girl with AD/HD much longer to fall asleep than a girl without AD/HD. In addition, the fallout from chronic sleep deprivation is that AD/HD symptoms tend to increase with fatigue and she may remain cranky and irritable. Recent research suggests a correlation between sleep disturbances and AD/HD in children. In fact, Provigil, a medication designed for treating sleep apnea and narcolepsy, is being used experimentally to treat AD/HD (Chervin et al., 1997; Corkum et al., 1998).

Bedtime rituals

Most parents complain that, because of how late their daughter actually falls asleep, they have no evening down-time for themselves without the child. Parent-child interaction after 10 PM often involves a power struggle between parents who are running on empty and a daughter who is defiant, overtired, and "needs" to tell you something "important."

Parents can help their daughter with AD/HD develop better sleep habits through establishing a well-defined bedtime ritual. Girls with AD/HD can rarely shift quickly from watching TV with siblings in the family room to turning the light off to go to sleep. These girls need extended time to "wind down" from the day. A warm shower or bath, followed by peaceful time in bed before the light is turned out, is often helpful. Having a story read to them, or, when they are older, reading to themselves, helps take their mind off the events of the day and prepares them for sleep. Girls who dislike reading may respond well to audiotapes of books or music before bed-time. They may also find that quietly playing the radio provides a sound screen that helps them tune out other sounds in the household while they fall asleep.

Socialization

While impaired social skills are not included in the DSM-IV diagnostic criteria for AD/HD, this symptom is very common among girls with AD/HD. Most girls with AD/HD have trouble initiating, developing, and maintaining friendships. They may have difficulty with a number of skills that affect social interaction, including give-and-take, conflict resolution, managing verbal expression, and difficulty picking up nonverbal cues.

One of the major stumbling blocks to successful peer relations lies in their inability to properly gauge their impact in a social interaction. Either they try too hard—intrusively pursuing idealized playmates while ignoring clear messages to "back off"—or they are demanding and controlling, so intent on satisfying their primary urges that they cannot be attuned to what their playmates are feeling. Either way, they may be viewed as insensitive to others' needs or, as their peers may describe it, "mean." And either way, the end result is that they push others away and end up alone, unable to see their role in these dramas, and tending to blame others for miscommunications. Unfortunately, this pushes others even further away.

Missing social cues

Interpersonal contact is always a challenge for the girl with AD/HD. Often, they are aware that their responses are different from those of their peers, but they don't know why. Emotions tend towards the extremes; they are intense, whether it is a feeling of anger, sadness, fear, silliness, or happiness. Once the feeling is aroused, it escalates quickly, often until the girl with AD/HD feels overwhelmed. At this point, it may be hard for her to calm down, even with adult guidance. The intensity of her feelings makes it difficult for her to attend to anything else in her world. "Anything else" includes the feelings of the child she is conversing with or the demands of the teacher. Because her own experience predominates, she may appear to be oblivious to the experience of others.

At other times, a girl with AD/HD may be so wrapped up in a barrage of external stimuli that it is nearly impossible for her to simultaneously remain in touch with her own inner state. Anger reactions may "sneak up on her" and her subsequent explosion may surprise her as much as it does the children around her. This sense of being ambushed by her own feelings is all too common for girls with AD/HD. Many girls cope by withdrawing to avoid experiencing this out-of-control feeling. Other girls barrel through, assertively acting on their feelings and being ambushed by the responses of others. Unable to recognize their impact, they are shocked by negative feedback.

The desire to belong

Girls who have difficulty reading social cues and reacting appropriately may benefit enormously from support groups where they can receive critical constructive feedback in an environment of acceptance and support. They may function better in more structured social activities where the rules are explicit. They also may function better in a one-on-one friendship with another girl. Sometimes relationships with younger girls or much older girls (such as a teenage babysitter or camp counselor) work better.

Because middle and high school are times of intense comparison, competition, and conformity, girls with AD/HD may find these years very difficult. Structured activities—art lessons, karate class, church groups, school clubs—may help them find a niche where they can stay out of the critical and competitive mainstream of high school, yet feel that they belong. Often, these girls find more acceptance in college and beyond, when their peers have matured beyond adolescent competition to greater tolerance, and they have a broader range of choices for friendships.

To summarize, the normative developmental tasks of early childhood are much more difficult to achieve, and are significantly delayed, in the girl with AD/HD. The result is that the girl with AD/HD wanders about in a world with less security and less predictability than her peers, unsure of others' reactions to her, and unsure of her own judgement because it so often betrays her.

School issues

The executive functions of the brain,—the management level that governs other functions—come to the fore in the school environment. A focus of recent research, it appears that ADHD children have chronic difficulties within the six clusters of executive functions. These functions include the critical abilities to:

1. Initiate, organize and prioritize tasks
2. Focus and sustain attention to tasks
3. Sustain alertness, effort and processing speed
4. Manage emotion and frustration
5. Access memory reliably
6. Monitor and control speech and behaviors (Brown, 1996).

The impact of AD/HD on executive functioning creates some of the most significant, and least understood obstacles to successful school performance (Denkla, 1989).

A girl with AD/HD may not have any difficulty understanding the material, but she may run into difficulty when she has to show what she knows. If she cannot organize her thoughts well enough to carry on a debate in class or create a plan for a long-term project, the end result will be that she does not perform well, regardless of how smart she may be. In fact, when a very smart girl turns in a seemingly haphazard report, it could easily be assumed that she's "just not trying" or "doesn't really care." Therefore, whether or not she knows the material, she will be penalized for her difficulties in initiating tasks and following through. This is a frustrating and demoralizing experience for a girl who knows the material, and, more importantly, knows she is trying as hard as she can.

Due to her organizational problems she may misplace her homework sheet, lose both of her pencils, and come to class without having finished reading the assigned chapter. She may have a chaotic binder, where papers stuffed in the front will be "put away later." One of the rumpled papers may be today's homework, appearing careless and messy due to poor handwriting and haphazard placement on the page.

It can be helpful to the student with AD/HD if her environment can be simplified, so that extraneous toys and books do not distract her. Help her to establish a storage system that she finds attractive and easy to use. Put together outfits the night before, allowing her to participate in selecting the garments. Choose your battles. This may mean allowing her to wear the same clothes for three days if she wants to. Try to embrace the fact that she is creating her own structured routine to help herself; while it doesn't follow your system, she ultimately needs to develop a system, however idiosyncratic, that works for her.

Planning difficulties

Planning difficulties might present themselves as:

- trouble managing long-term assignments
- not leaving enough time to eat breakfast and catch the school bus
- stopping in to "visit" with the guidance counselor three minutes before class begins

The ability to plan ahead plays a major role in the critical skills of managing time and setting realistic goals. In order to pursue a goal, the dreams of pride, reward, and appreciation must be put aside. The planning stage addresses and prioritizes the mundane and tedious steps that will ultimately lead to the goal. Make your daughter aware of the skills necessary for planning ahead. For example, if the family is going on an hour-long car trip, you can ask her, "How will you keep busy during the ride?" Brainstorm realistic solutions: "I know that you'd like to do some artwork, but paint is too messy for the car. Would you like to pack crayons or markers?" Giving her a choice of acceptable alternatives will allow her to feel empowered by making a decision about how to plan her experience.

Sequencing

Sequencing picks up where planning leaves off. After the goal is broken down into manageable smaller tasks, those tasks must be prioritized and placed in a sequence. Problems in sequencing emerge when a girl with AD/HD is trying to complete a list of things to do in an allotted amount of time, or remembering how to solve a multi-step equation in math. Sequencing is the skill most easily derailed by impulsive temptations. If her friends are stopping at the candy store after school, it will make it all the more difficult for her to remember that she needs to come straight home for her piano lesson. Instead of a punitive response, brainstorm ways she can remember to come home directly on Tuesdays, making her aware of the potential distractions that she must circumvent.

Memory

Remembering is a pervasive problem for the girl with AD/HD. It may be difficult for her to know when things are due, to bring materials back and forth between school and home, to remember to hand in assignments that may be in her binder, to memorize multiplication tables or other rote tasks, or to remember a sequence of steps to be followed. Sometimes, if she is not fully focused on the new information, she may not keep it in short term memory long enough to "file it." However, the response "I forgot" is often more about not being able to access and retrieve the information when she needs it.

Writing

The act of writing is a veritable minefield for many children with AD/HD: poor fine motor skills and difficulty persisting in motor activities make the physical act of writing uncomfortable. She may use too much pencil pressure, making her fingers ache with cramps and fatigue. The great discrepancy between the speed of her thoughts and the speed at which she can write makes her either leave out words in an effort to get the thoughts down, or forget some of her ideas while she struggles to print. For these reasons, a word processing computer program will greatly benefit AD/HD children of all ages. Difficulty organizing her thoughts, problems with word retrieval, and avoidance of a burdensome task make initiation of the writing assignment torturous. Finally, proofreading is too tedious for most girls with AD/HD; they can hyper-focus for a little while, but they may lose their motivation to finish.

You can assist your daughter in writing tasks if you allow her to brainstorm with you to "get over the hump" of how to begin. She may do well to dictate her thoughts to you so she doesn't have to struggle with handwriting and can focus on organizing her ideas. Early keyboarding skills are very important for girls with these types of difficulties. The new voice recognition software simplifies her task even more. She can dictate to her computer and then work on-screen to fine-tune her paper. In some schools, she can tape lectures or get notes taken by someone else to cope with note-taking, a notorious problem for students with AD/HD.

Test-taking

Girls with AD/HD may make numerous accidental errors, which are often described as "careless" by teachers and parents. These girls may have trouble finishing tests within the time limits because they are distracted, anxious, have difficulty retrieving the relevant information on demand, or are caught off balance by a novel test design. Extended time on tests, and taking tests in an alternate environment, separated from the class distractions, can help to reduce some of her difficulties. Oral exams can also be a boon because they allow her to demonstrate her knowledge without simultaneously struggling with the additional task of writing.

The classroom experience

Her cognitive style is not well suited for the classroom. Whether she works fast and sloppily, or painfully slowly and deliberately, she can't listen and take notes simultaneously, or feel comfortable during an open-book test; both require her to process two things at the same time. Craving novelty and being bored by repetition, she may be physically, mentally or emotionally uncomfortable in many classes. Nonetheless, she struggles to attend, despite a low frustration tolerance and difficulty sustaining effort. It is understandable that she sometimes seeks relief in a daydream.

Learning disabilities

In addition to the above issues, a significant number of girls with AD/HD have some type of learning disability. Even for the brightest girls, school can be a painful journey of underachievement. Much of their psychic energy is directed toward hiding their "differences," and not asking for help, leaving less energy to devote to required and leisure-time activities. They live with a pervasive sense of confusion and embarrassment. They know they are smart enough to be on top of things, yet they mysteriously underachieve, even when they are trying their hardest. This pattern could undermine even the most confident student making her doubt herself.

Reading

Dyslexia often co-occurs with AD/HD, however, even for girls with AD/HD whose reading skills are good, reading, especially if the content is not inherently interesting, can be incredibly difficult. Some reread the same passage over and over, struggling not to drift off. Some can hyper-focus for a couple of pages before they begin to skim, and then fall asleep from the effort. Some read quickly and superficially so that they can say they are "done," but have little comprehension or memory for what they've read. Some can only read in brief spurts; they prefer the "Newsweek" approach to current events: photos with catchy captions and a paragraph summarizing the issue. The only thing overtly noticeable to a teacher or parent is that these children read extremely slowly; the adults are then left to their own devices to interpret what they see. The interpretations chosen by authority figures have important repercussions for the ways these girls are approached.

They can hyper-focus on sentences in class. They become skilled scanners. Many children, longing to read stories, go to the library, enjoy storytime and take out several attractive-looking books. While they may touch them, open them, and study the covers, the books are usually returned unread. This is an area where children develop all sorts of compensatory techniques so that no one will know how painfully difficult it is for them to read.

When reading assignments, many girls with AD/HD find they have the best comprehension if they read it aloud to themselves. In fact, Vygotsky (1978) had suggested that many children find this kind of 'self-talk' comforting, organizing, and easier to focus on than listening or reading silently. It is a technique that works well for many girls with AD/HD and it is also, unfortunately, not acceptable in most classrooms.

Homework

Homework is the thorn in everyone's side: first, it is one of the most intense battles of the home front. Without the circumscribed structure of the classroom and the teacher's directions, homework may be perceived as a shapeless amoeba, with no clear beginning or end in sight. Kids are never completely sure of their assignments, or whether they have brought home all of the necessary materials. There is fear, dread, confusion, and sudden fatigue as they approach 5:00 PM—the hour they are expected to begin their homework. Thus begins the ritual of "circling the airport."

Like a pilot in a holding pattern, endlessly circling the airport, a girl with AD/HD may find seemingly endless excuses for "circling" her homework, before settling down to the dreaded task. As she prepares to "land," and begin her homework, she is distracted by tangential issues that allow her to procrastinate.

At 5:00 PM, in order to begin working, Sarah looks for a pencil and recognizes that the point needs to be sharpened, (regardless of how sharp it already is). She sees that the sharpener is full of wood shavings and needs emptying. She empties the sharpener over the wastebasket, but some shavings end up on the floor. She tries to brush each one under the desk with her hand. Finally, Sarah sits on the floor amidst piles of papers because her desktop is piled with so much clutter that she can't work there. Many of her papers are folded into small geometric figures; some of them are announcements from school that were meant for her parents. She unfolds one of these and thinks of bringing it downstairs to her mother, but first attempts to refold it along the original lines. By now, it is 5:30 PM and Sarah is no closer to landing than she was before.

There is no doubt that there is an element of active procrastination around homework. It is an activity that does not interest most children with AD/HD, or hold their attention, so it is always a struggle for them to apply themselves to it. You can help your daughter tame the homework monster by communicating specific expectations about the work process: "You can work for half an hour, take a 15-minute break, and then work for another half hour." You can help her divide up assigned reading so that she can do a little each day and not get overwhelmed. Take her to buy her favorite color highlighter. Above all, you can respect her limitations and acknowledge them, letting her know that you only expect her to try her best, and not to perform perfectly. For example, in helping her keep to her homework schedule, you can tell her, "I know that it's hard to keep track of the time while you're taking your break, so I'll check in and remind you when 15 minutes is up." Allowing her to set a timer empowers her even more to monitor herself.

The parent's role

A parent's job involves giving messages to their children, whether spoken, or unspoken, about how they should act and think. A girl who is inattentive, easily distracted, unmotivated, and impulsive will inevitably receive negative messages. Comments like, "Are you listening to me?", "Can't you finish one thing before you start another?", "Don't you understand that this is important?", "Don't touch that!", or even the repeated sighs of utter frustration, all contribute to her view of herself . As she begins to question her ability to judge a situation, self-doubt will increase. Eventually, these negative messages will be reinforced repeatedly and ultimately become internalized into her sense of self.

In search of self-esteem

Mothers have been shown to be more critical of their children with AD/HD than are fathers, suggesting that mothers, especially, need to become aware of the corrosive effect of long-term criticism (Barkley et al., 1990). But fathers are not necessarily more patient. Some studies have shown that children with AD/HD present less difficult and challenging behavior to fathers, with whom they may feel more intimidated or less familiar. Whether you are a mother or father, the best antidote to this undermining pattern of criticism is the tried and true advice: "Catch her being good!" It's important to consciously go out of your way to be warm, friendly, and supportive in order to counteract the frustration and negative reaction that you may be experiencing with your daughter. *How* you correct and *when* you correct make all the difference. Try to not let criticism be the first thing out of your mouth when you see her. When you correct, try to make it helpful rather than harsh. Praise her effort every chance you have.

The Catch-22

Society holds parents, especially mothers, directly responsible for their child's behavior. Indeed, until Alan Zametkin's ground-breaking study (Zametkin et al., 1990) demonstrated the neurological basis of AD/HD, the parents of hard-to-manage AD/HD children were looked upon with blame and disapproval. While respecting their daughter's differences, mothers also feel expected to achieve control of their daughter's behavior. This is a potentially impossible task that can leave parents exhausted, experiencing a wide range of emotions, including guilt, anger, compassion, fear, and rejection. Ultimately, the parents' feelings will define the family's attitude toward the problem, and this, in turn, will impact the efficacy of the interventions and their daughter's sense of self.

Even those mothers with a deep level of understanding of AD/HD, reach the end of their rope sometimes and say, "What's wrong with you? Why don't you ever listen?" Mothers with AD/HD themselves, whose frustration tolerance is often compromised, get especially annoyed with their daughter when they battle with an aspect of AD/HD that they dislike in themselves. Especially for undiagnosed parents with AD/HD, the multiple responsibilities and commitment of sending a child to school demands a level of organization that may push the limits of the envelope in terms of frustration. When a parent's need for personal space collides with an AD/HD girl's need to climb all over them, conflict will result. A good plan of action is to accept that this might happen, and to be prepared to leave the room for a few minutes. Let your daughter know that you need to take a break; it's a good strategy for anyone with AD/HD.

The good news

While we have identified characteristics of AD/HD that may prove problematic, many of these same tendencies have an adaptive side. The non-linear thinker who does not feel constrained by social conventions finds unusual ways of solving problems, and alternative ways of conceptualizing issues. Such children can become our most creative and independent thinkers. Girls with AD/HD may be more spontaneous, and may take risks that expand their experiences and help them reach goals. Their high energy level makes them tireless in pursuing a project of interest and dedicated and determined volunteers. Their symptoms can be reframed so that they don't just focus on their challenges, but appreciate themselves as unique and endowed with valuable strengths as well.

Protective factors

There are a number of factors that have been shown to make it more likely that a child with AD/HD will be successful. A supportive and intact family system can be attuned to and anticipate the needs of the girl with AD/HD. They can serve as strong and active advocates. AD/HD that is not complicated by any other co-occurring diagnoses also increases the likelihood of a good prognosis. Innate factors like temperament and genetic predispositions can greatly influence outcomes. In general, girls with AD/HD who grow up in a functional family with good communication skills, mutual respect, and no substance abuse or physical abuse, will have better outcomes. Children whose experiences are validated by their families are more likely to develop a strong sense of self-respect and be able to communicate their needs assertively.

The children of parents who practice consistent discipline with appropriate limit-setting also have a greater likelihood of a positive outcome (Biederman et al., 1995b). There may be a better outcome if neither parent has AD/HD, since the more members of a family with AD/HD, the higher the family stress level, overall. In addition, the more a family can learn about AD/HD, the more likely it is that they will learn to value individual differences, and the better they will be able to cope with AD/HD as a unit.

You always have the opportunity to change a negative into a positive: it is easy to catch your daughter misbehaving and disappointing you. However, it takes a bigger investment to "catch her being good." Letting her know that her behavior is what you hoped for will be the reinforcement she needs to perform the same behavior again. "You showed excellent judgement by finishing your homework before you talked to Sally on the phone." Frequent praise is a wonderful boost to self-esteem. Even if there haven't been any positive behaviors, you can reward her for inhibiting unwanted behaviors. For example, you might say, "I know that it was hard to sit quietly and wait to see the dentist. You did a great job!" Reinforcement also can take the form of an affectionate squeeze on the shoulder as you walk by, or a small material surprise that helps her remember that her efforts are appreciated is respected.

Self-Rating Scale to Help Identify Girls with AD/HD

The following is a checklist of possible manifestations of AD/HD in girls—a *self-report* questionnaire. This checklist is unique in that respect. Many of the issues and experiences for girls with AD/HD are "internal" and, therefore, not observable by others. Most AD/HD rating scales primarily focus upon observable behaviors as reported by others (parents and teachers). Because so many experiences of AD/HD are "internalized" for girls, we can only become fully aware of the issues with which they struggle by asking them directly.

This list has not yet had norms established, and, therefore should not be used for diagnostic purposes. If a girl finds that a significant number of these items relate to her, this does not necessarily indicate that she has AD/HD. However, if you find that she checks off a large number of issues, a professional evaluation may be appropriate. Ideally, this checklist should be reviewed together by the girl and a parent, teacher, or professional. This review can lead you to a discussion of important issues that she hasn't brought up before.

————✧∿∿∿✧————

AD/HD Self-Rating Scale For Girls

Mark each item with one of the code numbers below to show how much that feeling or behavior is part of your personal experience.

0 = that's not at all like me; that almost never happens to me
1 = that's a little like me; that happens to me but not very often
2 = that's a lot like me; that happens to me often
3 = that's just like me; that happens to me almost all the time

_____ 1. When most of the class has finished the assignment, I'm still working on it.

_____ 2. I daydream a lot.

_____ 3. Sometimes my mind wanders when I'm trying to listen to the teacher.

_____ 4. Sometimes I dread being called on by the teacher because I'm not sure what the question is.

_____ 5. I feel embarrassed in class because I don't feel as if I know what to do.

_____ 6. I feel uncomfortable in the school halls between classes.

_____ 7. I feel shy around my classmates.

_____ 8. Even when I have something to say, it's hard to raise my hand and volunteer in class.

_____ 9. I have trouble getting started on my homework.

_____ 10. I get in trouble for talking or giggling in class.

_____ 11. I bite my fingernails or chew on other things when I'm sitting in class or doing homework.

_____ 12. I interrupt other people, even when I try not to.

_____ 13. Sometimes other girls say I'm "mean" or "bossy."

_____ 14. I feel different from other girls.

_____ 15. I am a "tom boy."

_____ 16. I've had to go to the hospital to get stitches or for broken bones.

_____ 17. My handwriting is messy.

_____ 18. My hand hurts when I write for a long time.

_____ 19. I have arguments with my friends.

_____ 20. I accidentally bump into things like doorframes or table corners.

_____ 21. I make careless mistakes on tests.

_____ 22. Sometimes other girls don't like me, but I don't know why.

_____ 23. Sometimes, when I'm upset, I say things that I don't mean.

_____ 24. It's really hard for me to complete school projects.

___ 25. I read slowly and don't remember what I've read.

___ 26. I forget to bring in my homework or permission slips from home.

___ 27. I have trouble remembering all of the directions for an assignment.

___ 28. It's hard to concentrate on what I'm reading for more than a couple of minutes, unless it's something I'm interested in.

___ 29. Even when I've studied for a test, I can't remember the information when I'm taking the test.

___ 30. I wait until the last possible minute to start a project.

___ 31. I hand in my homework late.

___ 32. I forget to bring the right books home from school to do my homework.

___ 33. I don't get a chance to write down the homework assignment.

___ 34. I feel like I get my feelings hurt more than most girls.

___ 35. I feel ashamed a lot at school.

___ 36. I often feel like I want to cry.

___ 37. I don't feel as if I'm good at sports.

___ 38. I don't like to compete with other girls.

____ 39. Sometimes it feels as if I'm not good at any thing.

____ 40. It's hard to keep my desk neat.

____ 41. My room is very messy.

____ 42. My parents get mad at me for things I don't mean to do.

____ 43. I forget to do things my parents have asked me to do.

____ 44. I get a lot of stomachaches.

____ 45. I get a lot of headaches.

____ 46. I'm often late for school or other activities.

____ 47. I often miss the school bus.

____ 48. I have trouble getting up in the morning.

____ 49. My parents think it takes me a long time to get ready for school in the morning.

____ 50. In class, I'm distracted by what other students are doing.

____ 51. I get annoyed when someone is tapping their pencil or popping their gum near me.

____ 52. When I'm trying to do homework, I get distracted by little sounds, like a clock ticking or a bird singing outside my window.

____ 53. I wish my teacher knew how hard I try to do things right.

_____ 54. Sometimes my teacher seems mad at me, but I don't know what I did wrong.

_____ 55. My parents tell me I should try harder.

_____ 56. I often lose track of the time.

_____ 57. It's hard for me to sit still in class because I feel restless.

_____ 58. I feel best when I'm moving around—such as playing sports, running, or dancing.

_____ 59. I like to be active, not just sit around and talk like most girls.

_____ 60. My backpack is messy.

_____ 61. I don't like to go to a crowded store.

_____ 62. When I go somewhere with my parents, I wander off to look at something I'm interested in.

_____ 63. I spend a lot of time looking for things that I have misplaced.

_____ 64. My parents say I'm very creative.

_____ 65. When other girls are laughing at something that happens in class, I don't always get it.

_____ 66. Sometimes a girl will walk away from me and I don't understand why.

_____ 67. It helps if someone sits with me while I do homework, even if they're not helping me.

_____ 68. Sometimes I forget to eat.

____ 69. Sometimes I wait until the last minute to go to the bathroom.

____ 70. I never feel tired when my parents say its bed time.

____ 71. It usually takes me a long time to fall asleep after I get in bed.

____ 72. It feels as if I could play video games by myself for hours.

____ 73. I'm not always hungry at mealtimes.

____ 74. I often say I'll do something "in a minute" and then forget

____ 75. It's hard to go to sleep at night because my thoughts are racing in my brain.

____ 76. When I want to join a group, I don't know how to approach them.

____ 77. I feel bored a lot of the time.

____ 78. I don't like waiting in line.

____ 79. I often doodle or fiddle with something in my hand when I have to sit still.

____ 80. I feel bored and sleepy in class, but I wake up and feel energetic as soon as I stand up and move around.

____ 81. My friends say I'm "hyper."

____ 82. Bright lights and loud noises bother me a lot.

____ 83. I often lose things.

____ 84. I get teased for being "spacey."

ADDITIONAL QUESTIONS
FOR TEENAGE GIRLS

___ 1. It's very hard for me to keep track of home-work assignments and due dates.

___ 2. No matter how hard I try to be on time, I am usually late.

___ 3. I jump from one topic to another in conversation.

___ 4. I usually do assignments at the last minute, or turn assignments in late.

___ 5. My parents and teachers tell me I need to try harder in school.

___ 6. My parents say I'm irresponsible.

___ 7. My friends say I overreact sometimes.

___ 8. I feel anxious pretty often.

___ 9. Sometimes I feel moody and depressed, even for no reason.

___ 10. My moods and emotions are much more intense in the week before my period.

___ 11. I am quick to feel frustrated.

___ 12. It's hard for me to be patient.

___ 13. I wish my parents understood how hard high school is for me.

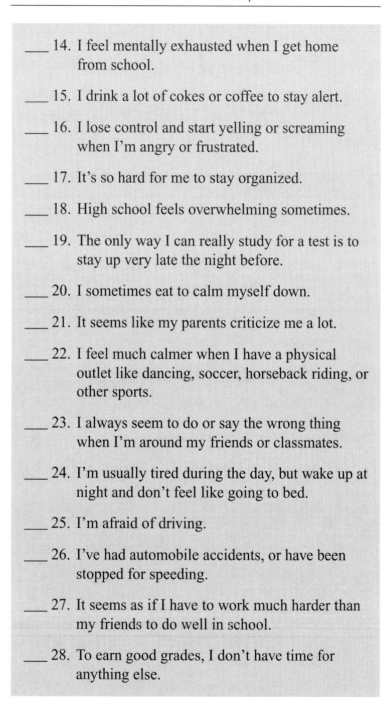

____ 14. I feel mentally exhausted when I get home from school.

____ 15. I drink a lot of cokes or coffee to stay alert.

____ 16. I lose control and start yelling or screaming when I'm angry or frustrated.

____ 17. It's so hard for me to stay organized.

____ 18. High school feels overwhelming sometimes.

____ 19. The only way I can really study for a test is to stay up very late the night before.

____ 20. I sometimes eat to calm myself down.

____ 21. It seems like my parents criticize me a lot.

____ 22. I feel much calmer when I have a physical outlet like dancing, soccer, horseback riding, or other sports.

____ 23. I always seem to do or say the wrong thing when I'm around my friends or classmates.

____ 24. I'm usually tired during the day, but wake up at night and don't feel like going to bed.

____ 25. I'm afraid of driving.

____ 26. I've had automobile accidents, or have been stopped for speeding.

____ 27. It seems as if I have to work much harder than my friends to do well in school.

____ 28. To earn good grades, I don't have time for anything else.

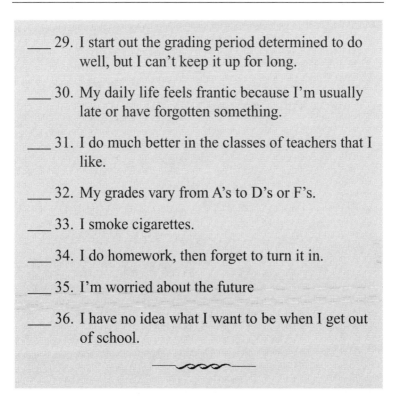

___ 29. I start out the grading period determined to do well, but I can't keep it up for long.

___ 30. My daily life feels frantic because I'm usually late or have forgotten something.

___ 31. I do much better in the classes of teachers that I like.

___ 32. My grades vary from A's to D's or F's.

___ 33. I smoke cigarettes.

___ 34. I do homework, then forget to turn it in.

___ 35. I'm worried about the future

___ 36. I have no idea what I want to be when I get out of school.

As for the other questionnaires throughout this book, this questionnaire should not be considered a diagnostic tool, but rather as a structured self-inquiry for girls when there is a concern about the possibility of AD/HD. When a girl answers "yes" to a majority of these questions, a professional evaluation may be advisable.

Chapter Five

The Preschool Years

Introduction

The preschool years encompass that time from roughly three to five years of age when a girl develops a sense of self and begins the process of mastery, self-determination, and venturing out into the larger world. It is a time of intense exploration and explosive changes, both physically and emotionally. It is also the time during which a girl acquires skills for beginning her academic career in the elementary school.

Diagnosing AD/HD during this period can be particularly problematic. One of the chief characteristics of this developmental stage is being active. Indeed, we tend to worry about the girl who is not engaging and exploring her environment, or who appears solitary or withdrawn. According to research on this subject, it is the preschooler's quality and degree of activity that is the crucial factor in distinguishing her from normal, naturally energetic, and exuberant peers. (Nichamin, 1972).

In addition to activity level, other behavioral clues can be helpful in evaluating the significance of any disruptive or inappropriate behaviors in a preschool girl. Is she aggressive? Does she have difficulty with transitions? Do certain textures or types of clothing bother her? Does she have difficulty falling asleep or staying asleep? Is she difficult to console, or is her reaction out of proportion to a given situation? Are tantrums unprovoked? Does she crave movement? Does she engage in risk-taking or dangerous behaviors? Is she highly impulsive? Are there problems with eating or toileting? Is she excessively withdrawn? Can she follow directions? Does the normal oppositional behavior of the "terrible twos" continue as she becomes three, four, and beyond?

DSM-IV subgroups apply to preschoolers

While not all preschool girls with AD/HD have problems in each of these areas, they usually fall into one of two subgroups designated in DSM-IV—the hyperactive/impulsive or the inattentive/distractible subtype. Many of the girls found in this latter subgroup may also appear to be shy and withdrawn, in addition to inattentive and distractible. We will discuss these girls in detail later in this chapter. However, it should be noted that many girls demonstrate characteristics from both subgroups and don't fall into any clear pattern. No matter what subgroup a girl may fall into, the important issue is to identify her problem behaviors early to prevent later academic, emotional, or social difficulties.

Studies of temperament have shown that early difficulties,

particularly the traits of being fussy, demanding, and difficult to manage, correlate with psychiatric difficulties during adolescence. However, prior to age five, family counseling to improve parent-child interactions seemed to be effective in preventing these psychiatric symptoms in adolescence (Terrikangas et al., 1998).

But how do we recognize AD/HD girls as toddlers or preschoolers? Let's look at each subtype, individually.

Hyperactive/Impulsive subtype

Jessica's mom knew early on that Jessica was different from her older sister. She had very advanced motor skills. She sat up early; she was pulling herself up at 7 months and walking by nine months. She was always on the go, and required little sleep. "Getting her to sleep at night and after nighttime feedings was very difficult. My husband spent hours rocking her on his shoulder." By age three, Jessica still wasn't sleeping through the night, and she had given up her daytime naps at 18 months. "She crawled out of her crib before she could walk and was always exploring or getting into things. While her running everywhere was appropriate as a young toddler, by age three we wanted more walking and less running."

Such girls may have trouble falling asleep at night or will wake up early in the morning. During these times, they frequently will get out of bed and play, or perhaps clean out their bedroom drawers, dumping all of the contents on the floor. In the morning, their rooms often are in disarray and the child may be found sleeping on the floor, in a closet, or under the bed.

Hyperactive preschoolers frequently may engage in dangerous activities, including climbing. One eighteen-month-old was found on top of the dining room table, literally swinging from the chandelier and jumping off onto the dog's back as he ran around the table! Preschoolers with impulsive risk-taking behaviors also may stand out in other ways. Jamie's mom thought that Jamie was just "accident-prone or perhaps more clumsy than other five-year-olds," but after her second broken bone and her third trip to the emergency room for stitches, Jamie's pediatrician questioned whether her risk-taking behaviors were out of the ordinary. In numerous studies, young children with AD/HD have been described as more accident-prone. Of all behavior variables, it was the amount of general activity that was most strongly related to accident frequency (Matheny, Brown & Wilson, 1971, 1972).

In some girls with AD/HD, hyperactivity may present as "hyper-verbal" or "hyper-talkative" rather in gross-motor terms:

Cathy talked early and her language development was precocious. However, she couldn't stop talking and commented on everything. While this appeared cute at first, it quickly became a problem for her peers and family members, who were often overwhelmed just trying to keep up. This type of chatter can be very disjointed and frequently off the target of the conversation. "While everyone else was discussing what he or she wanted to order at the restaurant, Cathy was talking about why Ronald McDonald has a red nose, or the present she wanted you to buy her for her birthday." Such girls may ask a million questions or chatter on endlessly. More than one mother has been heard to remark, "I wish she would just stop talking for one minute. She even talks to herself nonstop while playing alone."

Other girls may be active, but engage in more age-appropriate and acceptable activities:

Lang liked to play out of doors and was very athletic. She loved to climb trees and preferred to play with boys, but not always in a dangerous way. She was very coordinated and rode a two-wheeled bike without training wheels by her fourth birthday. She was usually cooperative and had a good relationship with her father. He enjoyed her "competitiveness" and "gutsy attitude." She could hit and throw a ball better than most boys her age, and was always sought after to play in their games.

Some girls at the hyperactive end of the AD/HD continuum are strong-willed and controlling and may have problems when playing with peers. Aimee was one such girl. Her mother characterized the situation in the following words: "All games must be her idea and played by her rules. She assigns the roles each are to take when playing, and she is usually the mother!" This behavior also caused problems between mother and daughter since Aimee always wanted to be in control. The home situation for such girls frequently may be described as more intense than in other families. It has been observed that mothers of such children tend to talk and play less with them. Mothers are also more frustrated and may tend to use more physical punishment with these girls.

———∿∿∿∿∿———

Teri was not only very hyperactive, she was also "bossy," and control was a major issue for her. Problems arose around eating and toilet training, as she tried to remain in control of all situations. These were only a few foods that she would eat, and these were mainly eaten as she got up and down from the table "a million times" during a meal. She refused to go to the potty and started pre-school in "pull-ups." As time progressed, her mother realized that Teri was "too busy" to stop and eat or use the potty. She also realized that these areas had become battlegrounds in the war for control. "In the end, I realized that the harder I pushed, or the more I yelled, the more firmly entrenched Teri became. Our days consisted of my yelling and Teri screaming or having one temper tantrum after another. My husband couldn't stand it. He blamed me for acting as "bad as Teri." He said I was constantly "getting down on her level" and "acting like a three-year-old myself." We argued a lot, but some days I couldn't disagree with his assessment of the situation. I didn't even like being around my own daughter."

———∿∿∿∿∿———

Dysphoria in preschool girls with AD/HD

Dysphoria is not included among the symptoms of AD/HD in DSM-IV, but in some girls with AD/HD, this issue of control can be carried to the extreme and a dysphoric (difficult, unhappy, and not easily satisfied) mood may dominate their interactions. Although these cases are not as prevalent as other types of AD/HD, such girls frequently cause the most distress for parents and teachers. Previously described in the literature as having a "difficult temperament," they can be seen clinically to go on to develop symptoms of AD/HD. More research is clearly needed to determine how commonly this presentation predates a diagnosis of AD/HD. Such girls are not happy with anything. They can be extremely frustrating to deal with since they are so difficult to please, and are often described as "not knowing what they really want" or as "insatiable."

―――――――⁓⁓⁓⁓――――――

Christine is typical of this subgroup. As an infant, she was extremely difficult. She had colic and cried a great deal. She was not adaptable and slept in "fits and starts." Early feedings did not go smoothly, and she seemed insatiable and difficult to please. "She didn't want her glass of orange juice placed here, she didn't want her glass placed there, and, in fact, she wanted apple juice." Dealing with these behaviors, her mother quickly became frustrated and depressed, often thinking that she was a failure as a mother. "Many days and nights were spent trying to soothe Christine. In the toddler phase, she entered the 'terrible twos' which never seemed to end." Christine could easily get out of control and her temper tantrums included falling on the floor or banging her head. Her parents became desperate and occasionally expressed that they wished they had never had a child.

Eating and toilet training issues also may be part of the picture. Christine became the child that you could never please. "She doesn't want what I have served for dinner (even if, yesterday, it was her favorite); she doesn't want her glass on the side of her plate; and maybe she doesn't even want that glass. She demands her favorite mug, which is in the wash, and refuses to drink unless she has it." Christine quickly became a tyrant as her parents desperately tried to "keep the peace." As her mother put it, "I feel that I'm being held hostage by a three-year-old."

―∞∞∞―

Inattentive/Distractible or "Shy/Withdrawn" subtype

In the late 1960's, researchers at NIH studying a population of preschoolers found that some girls with AD/HD presented behaviors that were the opposite of those expected—they were shy and withdrawn (Waldrop et al., 1978)

―∞∞∞―

Samantha is just such a preschooler. She had been a good baby, and was very placid and adaptable. She did not make great demands on her world as an infant. As she grew into a toddler, she did not readily join in with the other children, rather she watched from the sidelines. She tended to play by herself, over-focusing on one activity. She could play alone for hours when engaged in a favorite or familiar activity. However, when presented with multiple stimuli, she seemed overwhelmed and unable to focus on one thing. When given directions or tasks to perform, she tended to get distracted or "lost along the way," playing with something else that caught her eye. At times, when sent on an errand, she would get to the destination, but then forget what she had been sent for. Too many directions at one time overwhelmed her and she frequently reacted like a "deer caught in the headlights."

―∞∞∞―

Other parents have referred to these daughters as, "my child who stops to smell the roses." Some girls may be thought to have language delays or "auditory processing problems." Most parents and professionals rarely contemplate the diagnosis of AD/HD, but, unless the diagnosis is entertained, these girls can be dismissed and overlooked for years. They sit in the back of the classroom not causing any trouble, but they have no idea what is going on because their minds are somewhere else. They are perceived as "ditsy" or "not very smart," and many years are wasted as they grow to believe that they are not capable of achieving at the same level as others.

"Melinda began using a few words by the age of 18 months. Then at two years, she slowed down. As Melinda's world expanded into new experiences with nursery school, visits to the library, and swim time at the local pool, I realized that not only did Melinda continue to stare at strangers, she invariably was the last to participate in an activity. While all of her friends were bustling and shoving to be first, she hung back, reluctant, gazing out windows, smiling sweetly." Her mother took her for a speech and language evaluation as well as a hearing test. As expected, her hearing was normal, however, Melinda did demonstrate some difficulty with processing language, particularly when there was a lot of noise and commotion. She also had difficulty when she was given more than a single command. At the age of eight, Melinda was evaluated by a neuropsychologist who reported that she exhibited many characteristics of AD/HD. But, because she was not hyperactive, her parents had great difficulty convincing both the school and medical personnel of the diagnosis.

How do these girls behave in preschool?

Differences seen in the classroom for girls with AD/HD may stem from inattentive or impulsive behaviors which result in inefficient "cognitive styles." While no one girl may fall perfectly into a particular subtype, it has been shown that the problematic behaviors correlate with later competence and academic achievement. Studies of three-year-olds conducted by Richman and co-workers (1975) revealed a significant association between problem behaviors, poor rapport, and task orientation. The problem group had a tendency to be more active and fidgety and to show extreme moodiness. For boys, overactivity at age three, and for girls, shyness and difficulty separating, were shown to be correlated with behavior problems at school at age five (Coleman et al., 1977).

Hyperactive/Impulsive subtype

Hyperactivity in the classroom

The hyperactive and impulsive girls with AD/HD usually can be easily spotted in the preschool classroom. They have a great deal of energy and engage in lots of movement around the room. They never stay with one activity or play with one toy for any extended length of time. They go from activity to activity, but never really engage. When seated activities are required, these girls do not stay at the table for very long and show a considerable amount of "up and away" behavior. These girls tend to be "bossy" and more aggressive with other children. On the playground, they may engage in dangerous activities, such as scrambling to the highest rung on the climbing equipment, or into the branches of the tree which has been specified as "off limits." They may wander away and tend to run away from or ahead of the group. Field trips may be difficult, and these girls may need an adult assigned to just look after them.

In addition to having difficulty sitting still, hyperactive/impulsive girls with AD/HD may be talking, asking questions, or interrupting constantly. They like to dominate any situation and they require a great deal of attention. Indeed, they seek to be the center of attention and make it clear that they are not happy if they are not in that role. These girls are always seeking novel stimuli. However, when asked to recognize materials that have been presented before, they may act as if they have never seen them. They also tend to answer impulsively, giving fewer correct responses than their peers. They may demonstrate motor impulsivity, which also can be seen in their drawings. They tend to rush through craft activities and draw much faster than other children. These behaviors present problems for establishing early learning patterns, and cause difficulty with tasks such as learning, numbers, colors, and letters.

Naptime may be particularly difficult, as these girls need little sleep. Having long ago given up their naps at home, they have difficulty staying still in one place. They may prefer to roam around the room, sing, or talk through nap or quiet time, becoming a general disruption to others.

Negative classroom behaviors

At school, initially, the girl with difficult behaviors may not display all of the behaviors observed at home. However, she will eventually have difficulty meeting the demands of her class work. Perhaps she will have trouble starting an activity, or she may not want to finish when time is up, or when others are done with this activity. Power struggles will gradually appear in this setting, as well. These girls may cry more often and be more negative in general. They will have difficulty if offered too many choices, and can't easily make up their minds. They are inconsistent. On some days they may not want to nap, while on other days they may actually sleep for long periods.

Reactions may be out of proportion to the event, and these girls frequently have difficulty controlling their reactions. Angry displays such as foot stomping, arms crossed over the chest, and biting may become issues in the classroom. These girls may misperceive the behaviors of others, feeling that they have been slighted, or feeling that their space has been invaded when no slight was intended. Their behaviors tend to escalate and these girls may need physical restraining or frequent "time-outs" away from the group in order to calm down. Moods and responses are unpredictable and change quickly. These girls may be perfectly delightful while on a field trip and only have difficulty when it's time to leave.

Inattentive/Distractible or "Shy/Withdrawn" subtype

Typical classroom behaviors

The girls who are shy and withdrawn may look very different from hyperactive/ impulsive girls in preschool. Their behaviors may isolate them from the other children and they frequently may be seen observing the others from the sidelines of the group. They appear as daydreamers and can be easily distracted from a task. They have difficulty transitioning from one task to another and may always be one step behind the others. They frequently may misplace or lose mittens, hats, coats, and even their shoes.

These girls often appear to prefer solitary play, and frequently overfocus on an activity. They become lost in what they are doing and are unaware of what is going on around them. At times, they seem confused. Naptimes and clean-up times are difficult because of the transitions involved. These girls are not very adaptable and have difficulty with new routines or personnel in the classroom. Field trips present problems because of the break in routine and the new surroundings.

Auditory processing and language skills

Ability to follow directions and auditory processing may be delayed for these girls. They may have difficulty expressing themselves and/or actually have language delays. They may have difficulty paying attention to a story read to them, and may not be able to relate clearly what went on at home or during the day at school. Visual clues tend to help orient them, and the need for sameness is essential.

Making the diagnosis

Many of the behaviors described in this chapter are perfectly appropriate for infants and toddlers up to the age of two. So how can you tell if there is a problem and that the behaviors you are seeing are more than developmental? Making a diagnosis of AD/HD in children in this preschool period remains a controversial issue, but one that needs to be addressed if we are to avoid the negative effects on self-esteem, relationships, and academic potential that multiply as the years progress without a proper diagnosis.

Problem behaviors may be more prevalent at home

Younger children with AD/HD tend to exhibit higher activity levels than older children with AD/HD, and their behaviors may be more situational. Behaviors also may not be as pervasive, and may occur more at home than at school. Mothers frequently blame themselves when their child acts out only at home. They feel that they cannot handle the situation and that they are the cause of the problem. Many feel that if they only had better parenting skills, things would be better.

While counseling to improve parent-child relations does improve the situation, this does not mean that the parent was the cause of the problem. Frequently, we only see the problems at home when a girl is younger because this is the setting in which she is most comfortable being herself.

This does not mean that a real problem does not exist. Remember that true AD/HD is a neurobiologic condition and is not caused by poor parenting. Although poor parenting skills can make the problem worse, as we have seen, they are not the cause of the problem. Being a parent is a difficult and time-consuming job, at best. Being the parent of a daughter with special needs can be extremely challenging and frustrating, as well as exhausting.

Seek the help of professionals

The most important first step toward obtaining a diagnosis is seeking the help of professionals trained in working with young children. While many professionals are well trained and have experience with elementary-school-aged boys, very few have experience or expertise in diagnosing preschoolers or girls.

Gathering information from others

Gathering information from preschool teachers, daycare providers, and babysitters also will be helpful. These professionals have experience in dealing with many children in this age group. This may be your first or second child. If your other children did not have AD/HD, it may be difficult for you to decide if there really is a problem.

Gathering information within the family

AD/HD often runs in families. Talk with other family members. Has anyone else had the same problems as a child? Have other siblings, cousins, nephews, or nieces been diagnosed with AD/HD or learning disabilities? Does either parent have symptoms of AD/HD, diagnosed or undiagnosed?

Consult with your pediatrician

Talk with your pediatrician. He or she should be able to discuss your child's development up to this point, and any risk factors related to the pregnancy and/or family history. However, as many pediatricians are not trained in the diagnosis of AD/HD in children this young, it is important to convey your concerns and assess if they are being seriously addressed. Don't feel that your pediatrician has all the answers, or that you are being disloyal for seeking help elsewhere. It is still rare that a pediatrician recognizes AD/HD, especially without hyperactivity, in a preschooler.

Seek "early identification" programs

All school systems must, by law, have programs to identify children "at risk" for behavior or learning problems. This is another avenue that you may wish to pursue. Head Start and early identification programs in your area should offer screenings and evaluations.

Using AD/HD questionnaires

AD/HD is a diagnosis based on history and observed behaviors (symptoms). There is no specific test for AD/HD, and the disorder cannot be ruled in or ruled out by looking at a child's behavior in only one setting. Ask questions and read as much as you can. Be aware that the diagnosis exists in preschoolers, and learn how it presents in girls. This is the only way that you will be able to ascertain if your daughter, student, or patient has AD/HD. Using questionnaires and asking questions, such as the ones offered at the end of this chapter, are the two best ways for gathering information to make the proper diagnosis. Questions, such as the ones at the end of this chapter, may be very useful in alerting you to the possibility that there is a problem.

Importance of direct observation

Younger children frequently do better in free play situations, and it may not be until structured activities are required that any problems are observable. Direct observations in a structured play situation should be conducted prior to making the diagnosis of AD/HD. If this is not feasible, then a discussion with the girl's preschool teacher or caretaker may suffice.

Importance of physical exam and testing

A physical examination, vision and hearing tests, a neurodevelopmental screening, and psychoeducational testing should be performed on all girls for whom the diagnosis of AD/HD is being entertained. Doing this can rule out other conditions that may be contributing to the presenting symptoms. In addition, psychological testing can help rule out specific learning differences and aid in defining learning strengths.

Handling the situation

Once a preschool girl has been diagnosed with AD/HD, there are several positive steps to take to make things better at home and in school. The most important first step is seeking help. Girls with AD/HD are more difficult to handle in many settings. Whether the girl is hyperactive, shy, irritable or stubborn, parents and teachers need to become aware of how to assist her in becoming better integrated into a program and relating positively to others.

- Educate yourself about AD/HD
  Parents and teachers may need to become more knowledgeable about the disorder, its manifestations, what works, and what doesn't work by reading many of the good books available on this subject. We recommend, *Sourcebook for Children with Attention Deficit Disorder: A Management Guide for Early Childhood Professionals and Parents by* Clare Jones (1991, The Psychological Corporation).

- Remain positive
  Parents, caretakers, and teachers need to remain positive. Remember it is the girl's *behaviors* that are the problem, and not the girl herself. Many girls

grow up feeling that they are "bad," "not very
smart," or that there was "something wrong with
them" because of the negative comments they've
heard throughout their lives.

- Learn parenting skills
  It is important to read about AD/HD and how to
  parent a difficult child. Attend parenting classes or
  seek the help of a therapist or family counselor
  to assist you.

- Behavior management techniques
  Learning new behavior management techniques is
  extremely important. They can help you better deal
  with your daughter's behaviors, and help address or
  eliminate problem situations such as transitions.

- Choose appropriate activities
  Working with an expert can help you choose appropriate activities for your daughter/student based on
  her developmental level. Appropriate activities can
  reduce her frustration and will help her build confidence.

Dealing with out-of-control behaviors or temper tantrums

Fewer choices

Girls with AD/HD should be offered fewer choices to avoid
power struggles and tantrums. If these behaviors do arise,
they should be managed with firmness and consistency.

Time-out

A brief time-out, or simply ignoring the behavior may be appropriate ways to handle tantrums. Time-out works by removing the girl, who is out of control, from the situation and allowing her time to process and calm down. This technique, when used consistently and calmly, can be used with girls as young as two. The period of time-out should be kept brief and be used consistently with few words or explanations. The rule of thumb is one minute of time-out per year of age. The girl, herself, may even see the value in the practice.

Holding

When a girl with AD/HD is extremely out of control, or she is a danger to herself or others, the issue of holding often arises. Using this technique, the adult in charge of the situation will hold the girl tightly until she has calmed down. Girls often are able to tell you if they are "okay" or that they no longer need to be held. Time-out also may work if the girl is sufficiently in control at the time or once she has calmed down. Physical punishment or spanking is rarely appropriate under any circumstances.

Avoid power struggles

As one mother put it, "One of the most important lessons we have learned is the art of compromise. I have also had to learn to make a demand and wait when Carla is in one of her stubborn moods. Her overall goal is to please, but she has to reconcile how she can please me and not feel as though she has 'lost.' I usually give her a choice and then back off so she can decide to do the right thing."

"We had been using time-out at home for some time. Initially when Mary's behaviors were out of control, we would consistently remove her to time-out. Over several months, she became used to it. Eventually all I needed to say was 'I think you need a time-out, now,' and she would go over to a little bench we had set up in the family room, sit down and look at one of her books. When she came back to the situation she was usually calmer and more cooperative. One day, when I was visiting her nursery school class, I noticed that Mary was becoming excited during a game of musical chairs. She was laughing and starting to touch and pull on the other children. I could see things escalating and getting out of control. All at once, Mary ran from the group and sat in a big beanbag chair and held up a book to cover her face. I was amazed. She was giving herself a 'time-out' just like at home. After a few minutes, she seemed calm and rejoined the group when invited. I was so proud of her and glad we had been using the technique at home."

Anticipate and plan

In working with a girl with AD/HD, it is also important to anticipate difficult situations. Difficult situations may include:

- Transitioning to bed
- Meal-time
- Toilet training
- Playing with others
- Getting along with siblings

Bedtime issues

Bedtime may precipitate many problem behaviors. For some girls, bedtime represents a time of separation from parents or older siblings. This issue needs to be addressed with understanding and consistency. Bedtime rituals, firm limit setting, and constant reassurance are usually enough to address this problem. Allowing a child to stay up until she is tired or ready for bed does not address the issue, and usually results only in a tired and cranky child the next day. Many children demand that their parents remain in the room or lie down with them until they fall asleep. Some prefer to fall asleep in the parents' bed or come into the parents' bed during the night. Neither of these solutions addresses the issue of separation or control, and is therefore not adequate.

"I now recognize that Keisha just does not need as much sleep as her older sister. I allow her to stay up later, in her room, and play until I come up and turn out the light. Putting her in her own room has helped, because now we are not worried that she will wake her older sister or baby brother. We also have bought her a set of headphones and she loves to listen quietly to music or stories on tape. These also work great on long car rides."

For girls who need little sleep, playing quietly in their room or listening to tapes of music or stories may be an option. For girls who awaken and get up during the night, it is important to offer protection from dangerous situations, such as going outdoors alone, climbing on high objects, or getting into the kitchen near the stove, etc. This may be accomplished by locking the kitchen door, setting up a gate in the bedroom doorway, or double-locking the front door of the house. Alarm systems are now relatively inexpensive and can be set up with motion detectors and an alarm that sounds when a door or window is opened. Bright girls with AD/HD are very creative. Parents just need to be more creative in finding solutions.

"Jessica had started waking up very early, before 6 AM on the weekends. Gone were the days when she would entertain herself in her room, playing and looking at her toys. She would get up, go downstairs, eat food, and make a mess. After a string of what I thought were impossible days, one when she had climbed up on a chair, opened the freezer, gotten out ice cream, left the freezer open and gone out on the back deck to eat the ice cream, we decided we needed to do something. My husband sawed her bedroom door in half (like an old 'Dutch' door) and we put a lock on the bottom half. When Jessica was safely in her room and had been kissed good night, we locked the bottom half. We repeated, as she had been told previously, that if she needed us, all she had to do was call, and that in the morning she could have a 'treat' with breakfast if she stayed in her room. It worked like a charm, and we felt better knowing that Jessica was safe!"

Toilet training

Toilet training easily can become an area for confrontation and control. In general, girls are trained more easily and are developmentally ready sooner than boys. However, if a girl is not ready, she should be allowed more time. If wetting occurs because of lack of awareness, frequent reminders or scheduled visits to the bathroom may help. Early accidents as a result of not paying attention to the need to go to the bathroom are common. However, they can lead to embarrassment and cause a girl to not want to leave home. Bedwetting is seen more frequently in children with AD/HD and may be an issue for girls as well. Handling this situation with caring and concern is the best approach.

───✺───

"Toilet training had been late for her sister, so I was not worried when Jessica started pre-school in pull-ups. As time progressed, however, I realized that she used pull-ups because it was convenient and she did not have to stop what she was doing to go to the bathroom. I put her in underwear and told her she would earn a sticker every time she used the potty. Within a week, she was happy and no longer even asking for stickers. Bowel movements have been more difficult, but again the stickers worked very well. The last hurdle will be to not wear pull-ups to bed."

───✺───

Mealtime issues

Control issues and behavior problems also may arise around mealtime. Some girls have difficulty stopping an activity in order to eat. Others may have issues with food textures and preferences. It's best to deal with sensory issues with an occupational therapist as part of a total treatment program for sensory sensitivity. Control and attention issues need to be addressed separately with limit setting and a behavior management system—a system that rewards appropriate behaviors, such as tasting a variety of foods or eating small amounts of a non-preferred food, with an extra serving of a preferred food.

―✥―

"By the time Carrie was three, she would only eat macaroni and cheese, applesauce, and yogurt. I was concerned about her nutrition, and when our pediatrician told me after a check-up that she was slightly anemic, I was really worried. Because of some other sensory hypersensitivity (Carrie didn't like labels on her shirts and would only wear soft sweat pants), he recommended we see an occupational therapist. She explained to me about problems with hypersensitivity, and we began a program to gradually increase what Carrie would eat. It took several months, but by being consistent and offering her rewards and her favorite foods as treats, we gradually added to the foods that she would eat. She eventually started eating hamburger, soups with chicken and vegetables (cut up in small pieces but pureed at first), and other mashed fruits. We continued occupational therapy and a desensitization program. Eventually the pieces of food she could tolerate became bigger."

―✥―

Remember Teri and her mother from earlier in this chapter? They were also having difficulty in the area of control around toilet training and mealtime. Well, their story also has a happy ending.

―✥―

"With the help of our family therapist, I set up a behavior program to address these issues with Teri. I decided to pick one behavior and try to focus on

changing it rather than constantly trying to change everything at once. I chose getting up from the table before she had finished her food as the behavior to target. It was difficult, but with constant reminders and smaller portions, she gradually could eat a meal at one sitting. From here, we moved on to going into the bathroom and sitting on the toilet. I realized these were small steps, but we were now making progress."

Social interactions

Playing with others, such as siblings or peers, also can be a problem area. Rough play may lead to over-stimulation and problems with stopping an activity. Play dates with only one or two other children may need to be arranged. Planned, supervised activities usually work out better than unsupervised or unstructured playtimes. The child with AD/HD needs to know the limits. Acceptable, as well as unacceptable, behaviors should be reviewed beforehand. Large gatherings such as birthday parties can be difficult, and behaviors usually deteriorate as excitement escalates. Planning a smaller get-together is usually more successful.

Girls who are shy and inattentive also may find large groups overwhelming.

"When participating in preschool birthday parties in the neighborhood, Melissa always seemed overwhelmed. Instead of showing excitement by plowing into the games and candy like the other children, she would cling to me and refuse to get off my lap or unwrap herself from my leg. She would smile, but refuse to take her 'goody bag,' and seemed on the 'verge of tears' the rest of the time. Other mothers commented

on her distress and I was worried that she would soon not be invited at all. I was also dreading her birthday in the fall. When that time came, we decided just to invite another quiet little boy and girl, who were her friends. We set up a video in the family room and had cake and ice cream without singing 'Happy Birthday.' Her friends only stayed for about an hour and all seemed to go well. Melissa even seemed genuinely unhappy that they were leaving when it was over."

Girls with AD/HD may have difficulty playing gently with younger siblings, especially infants and toddlers. Often they irritate older siblings by invading their space or tagging along. It is important that off-limit areas (such as older siblings' bedrooms) be set up and strictly enforced. It is important to also try to avoid always assigning the role of "babysitter" to older siblings. This may cause them to resent their little sister. However, older siblings may be called into service on occasion on a contractual basis, once they are old enough to understand how to properly supervise and deal in a helpful way with their younger sister with AD/HD. Preschool girls like to be helpful around a baby. Assisting in diapering or bathing by fetching needed equipment or playing in the tub with a younger sibling, while supervised, may meet this need.

Multi-modal treatment approaches
Medication for preschoolers

For girls with a high level of hyperactivity or impulsivity, or who are dangerous to themselves or others, the use of medication, even at this young age, may be indicated. Aggressiveness and uncontrolled temper tantrums may negatively affect family and/or peer relationships, and for these girls the use of medication can be a lifesaver. Research has shown that medication at the proper dosage can decrease activity levels, improve compliance, and improve mother-child interactions (Barkley, 1988). The stimulants and other medications used to treat these disorders will be discussed in a later chapter. We will not focus on them here, other than to say that they have been tested, work well, and can be used safely with children in this age group.

Other therapies

Additional therapies may be necessary to address motor or language delays. The girl with AD/HD already may be experiencing learning difficulties based on her cognitive style; the additional burden of other developmental delays may further complicate the situation. An occupational or physical therapist and/or a speech pathologist may be necessary as adjuncts to her educational program to deal with language delays, hyper-sensitivities or sensory integration dysfunction, and fine or gross motor coordination difficulties or delays. Placement in special education or programs for children "at-risk" for learning difficulties may be appropriate in order to avoid problems in the future.

Classroom placement

Proper classroom placement also is important. Girls with AD/HD do better in a structured setting, but it is always important to seek out as good a "match" between teacher and student as possible. Placement should take into account the individual needs of each girl. This includes such issues as activity level, disorganization, fine and gross motor development, and need for structure and creativity. The teacher's attitude and education regarding learning differences, the school's philosophy, and individual teaching styles all need to be taken into consideration. Classrooms, as well as home, should be childproofed to protect the impulsive preschool girl.

Conclusion

One of the most consistent characteristics of AD/HD is its inconsistency. Coupling that with the normalcy of some of these characteristically AD/HD-behaviors before the age of three makes AD/HD difficult to diagnose in the preschool years. Having said this, however, it is imperative that we begin to do a better job of diagnosing AD/HD in preschool populations. In this chapter, we have discussed several separate presentations of AD/HD in girls of this age group. But, life is rarely so simple or clear cut. Your daughter, student, or patient may be displaying symptoms of all these types. Diagnosticians have also observed this phenomenon, and have resolved this issue by designating a "Combined Subtype" of the disorder. However, more research is needed on girls with difficult temperaments or dysphoria. We also need to look at the shy/withdraw preschoolers and better document their difficulties within the subgroup of the inattentive/distractible. And what of the girl whose early problems don't result in academic difficulties until later elementary years or middle school? What of the young girl who has frequent mood swings, is overly sensitive, or who cries often and easily? Does she later go on to have depression as well as AD/HD? We need answers to all of these questions.

The importance of early diagnosis

The early diagnosis of AD/HD is important for several

reasons. Early diagnosis leads to earlier treatment and intervention programs. Such early intervention programs can prevent many secondary problems from developing. Early diagnosis allows for the establishment of good habits and patterns, sets up positive relationships, and encourages the development of better parenting skills. Your daughter also will feel better about herself.

There is much that we can do to help girls with AD/HD live happier, more satisfying lives, and the sooner we start the better. Preschool is NOT too early. Much of the damage to self-esteem and interpersonal relationships is already well under way by the age of seven. If you feel that your daughter or student is experiencing difficulty, seek an evaluation or professional guidance. You and she will be glad that you did!

QUESTIONS TO ASK YOURSELF ABOUT YOUR PRESCHOOLER

(This list was designed to raise your level of awareness and aid you in asking the right questions. We encourage you to take a look at your preschool age daughter, student, or patient with these typical behaviors in mind, and to seek further evaluation if your suspicions are aroused by the following questions.)

Consider your preschooler

☐ Is she restless or overactive?

☐ Does she run instead of walk?

☐ Does she have trouble sitting still?

☐ Is she always up and on-the-go?

☐ Is she squirmy and fidgety?

☐ Does she have a short attention span? (10-15 minutes is average for this age.)

☐ Does she have difficulty concentrating on or playing with one toy for any length of time?

☐ Does she have difficulty listening to a story being read to her?

☐ Does she engage in dangerous activities?

☐ Does she not show appropriate fear?

☐ Does she have frequent accidents (stitches, cuts, bruises, broken bones, or visits to the ER)?

☐ Does she "bully" other children?

☐ Is she "bossy"?

- ☐ Does she kick, bite, or hit others?
- ☐ Does she have difficulty sharing toys?
- ☐ Does she often stare into space?
- ☐ Is she a daydreamer?
- ☐ Does she give up easily?
- ☐ Does she often stand on the sidelines and watch before joining in a group activity?
- ☐ Does she worry excessively?
- ☐ Does she prefer to play on her own (solitary play)?
- ☐ Is she fearful or afraid of new situations?
- ☐ Does she talk very little in public?
- ☐ Does she have delayed speech or language skills?
- ☐ Does she have difficulty expressing herself?
- ☐ Does she misplace or lose belongings?
- ☐ Is she irritable?
- ☐ Is she miserable or unhappy?
- ☐ Does she cry often and easily?
- ☐ Does she have temper tantrums?
- ☐ Is she fussy or overly particular?
- ☐ Does she blame others?
- ☐ Do others like her?
- ☐ Does she destroy toys?
- ☐ Is her toilet training delayed (beyond three years)?
- ☐ Does she still wet or soil herself, although she's "trained"?
- ☐ Does she rarely nap or rest quietly, even when tired?

Chapter 6

The Elementary School Years

To best appreciate the special challenges faced by elementary school girls with AD/HD, it is helpful to view them against the backdrop of typical development for this age group. In most cultures, after age five, children are no longer restricted to the home or to settings where they are closely monitored by caregivers. Instead, these young children are challenged to become increasingly responsible for their own behavior in a variety of new social contexts. To succeed within this framework of greater autonomy, the elementary-school-age child must take over some of the supervisory responsibilities that have previously been the domain of adults. Many children begin to learn to plan ahead, prioritize, organize, and monitor their own behavior during this stage of development.

What is normal development?

The defining developmental characteristic of this stage is greatly increased cognitive capabilities—the ability to think logically and flexibly, to keep track of more than one thing at a time, to perform tasks independently, to formulate goals and resist the temptation to abandon them (Piaget, 1929). Piaget believed that the key to these increased cognitive capacities lay in the crystallization of a higher form of thought that he called "concrete operations." This new level of reasoning helps a child make her physical world more predictable. For example, when a child begins to understand that she can pour water from a tall pitcher into a short bowl and the total volume of water remains unchanged, she can impose structure on the unknown. Each of these little discoveries lessens the amount of uncertainty she feels about the world, and allows her to venture forth with more confidence.

With the foundations of trust, separation, and individuation falling into place, the elementary school girl becomes freer to focus her energies on school challenges, both academic and interpersonal. School begins to occupy a central role in her life, and provides an abundance of new stimuli from teachers and peers. The skills necessary to process all of this new information are being learned continuously during this period. As little girls play together, usually in pairs, they create a detailed context in which they can engage in complex verbal negotiations. This play-acting, whether centered on Barbie's exploits or a take-off on the Little Mermaid, helps them to understand much about the give-and-take necessary for successful communication. They begin to learn to relate appropriately to a wide range of adults and children, using information gained in one situation, which they will attempt to generalize to the next.

A fact easily forgotten is that development is notoriously uneven at this time—both among the characteristics of a given child and between children across a given characteristic. While this fact is widely known, in the face of all of these emerging abilities, it is not surprising that adults tend to forget that these wide developmental differences are normal. While the realities of uneven development may be comfortable for parents with precocious children, they can be anxiety provoking for those whose children may lag behind. Parents can be seduced when they see flashes of higher cognitive understanding in their daughters; they may be moved to raise their overall expectations. These young girls try to stretch in order to comply, eager to earn positive feedback. This is the essence of the daunting work of the elementary school years.

How AD/HD complicates the elementary school years

Learning to generalize from a specific situation to other similar situations is necessary for problem solving in life. While a girl with AD/HD may grasp the constancy issues in pouring half the container of milk into her thermos, she may not be able to generalize that event to any other situation. Often, the novelty of a new situation can provide imbalance that may derail the fragile mastery of skills that she has achieved.

Michelle is an 8-year-old girl with AD/HD who joined the Brownies. Since this is her first extracurricular group activity, Michelle finds their Tuesday afternoon outings both scary and exciting. Her troop sometimes returns from their local outings earlier than expected, and the girls run around when they return. While parents have been told to arrive at 5:00 PM, Michelle has a hard time waiting patiently, and she is often crying by the time her mother arrives. Her mother has solved this problem by suggesting that Michelle call her as soon as they return to the community center. When Michelle calls, her mother does her best to pick her up immediately. Michelle and her mother succeeded in their plan on two different occasions, and both mother and daughter were pleased with the results.

When the troop went to the nature preserve, they took a school minibus instead of walking, and the bus returned them to the elementary school. Michelle was confused, but she tried to wait with several other girls after most had been picked up. As the remaining girls were picked up, Michelle became increasingly frantic, not understanding why her mother didn't arrive. At 5:00 PM, her mother arrived at the community center and was directed to the school. When she arrived at the school at 5:07 PM, Michelle was with the leader, crying hysterically. Just enough variables had changed to rob Michelle of her sense of control. Reacting with the emotional intensity of many girls with AD/HD, she felt frightened and abandoned.

When Michelle calmed down a half-hour later, she said she was going to drop out of the Brownies. As her mother tried to reason with her, Michelle put her fingers in her ears and sang. Her mother felt very guilty and offered to buy Michelle a new Beanie Baby.

These scenarios reflect a common pattern between mothers and their daughters with AD/HD. The mother teaches her daughter a skill; the daughter demonstrates learning of skill, but then an instance arises where daughter does not use skill, and both mother and daughter are at a loss to explain why. Both mother and daughter feel annoyed and disappointed; the sequence of events ends with mother feeling guilty for having unreasonable expectations of her daughter, and with daughter feeling guilty for failing her mother. Because of the gender-determined focus on the connection between mother and daughter, the disruption of their relationship exacerbates the girl's simple failure to use a skill.

Misleading behaviors

Carol Gilligan (Gilligan, 1982) has highlighted the gender differences between girls' and boys' definitions of moral behavior. She explains that girls generally define morality in terms of conflicting responsibilities rather than the more male-valued terms of competing rights. In other words, a girl may feel that winning a game also leaves her opponent feeling sad, and she may perceive those as conflicting outcomes that may create anxiety for her. The comfort level of the relationship between the friends may have greater importance to her than her own achievement, which threatens to place her *above* her friend and disrupt their mutuality. On the other hand, a boy may be thrilled to be the winner, feeling that he has worked to earn his superior position over his opponents, as long as he knows he has played by the rules.

However, AD/HD makes it difficult for girls to examine and remain aware of their conflicting responsibilities simultaneously. It is difficult for the girl with AD/HD to distinguish what feels urgent to her versus what may be deemed most important, in the big picture, by others. Therefore, it may appear that these girls subscribe more to the school of competing rights, and aren't as guided in their behavior by interpersonal connection. In fact, they simply may be responding to the matter that has the greatest inherent interest for them at the moment. Ultimately, girls without AD/HD may feel that girls with AD/HD are not playing by the same set of rules.

The challenge of connectedness

Carol Gilligan uses the metaphors of the web and the ladder to illustrate the distinction between girls' and boys' relationships. The web can symbolize interconnectedness, as well as entrapment; the ladder suggests an achievement orientation, as well as individualistic and hierarchical thinking. For the girl with AD/HD, impulse-driven responses are often similar to the achievement-oriented responses more typical of boys. The cost of her gender-inconsistent responses may be peer rejection, for which she can see no logical explanation. She may be left with less predictability and security than her peers, steeped in the sense that she can't really trust her judgement because it so often betrays her.

In a different type of self-monitoring failure, a girl can be so hyper-focused on her own experience that she may be ambushed by the responses of others.

Penny began to braid the hair of Mary Ann, who sits in front of her in class. Initially, Mary Ann accepted this and thanked Penny. With this positive reinforcement, Penny's spirits soared as she kept undoing the braid and rebraiding it. Soon, Mary Ann asked Penny to stop. Penny, giddy because she was connecting with another child in a seemingly intimate way, didn't really process the request. If anything, there was generally higher stimulation in Mary Ann's excited response. Mary Ann became increasingly annoyed with Penny, until she finally turned around and yelled, "Don't touch me anymore!" Penny, feeling completely ambushed by Mary Ann's reaction, started to cry. Since she was unable to assess her impact on the situation, she was shocked by Mary Ann's negative response, which seemed to come out of nowhere.

It is easy to see that Penny has yet to achieve the developmental skills that would allow her to simultaneously monitor her own experience as well as Mary Ann's. As a result, she is unable to make the chaotic world of social interactions any more predictable for herself at this point in time. She learns that one of the risks of relationships is ambush.

What the subtypes of AD/HD look like in elementary school girls

Hyperactive/Impulsive subtype

When I was called in to evaluate Jan in first grade, her teacher voiced concern that Jan simply could not sit still at circle time, despite various teacher interventions. The teacher, Mrs. Leeds, felt that Jan was bright and understood what was expected. She didn't find Jan to be oppositional, but was at a loss to explain her behavior. When I was alone with Jan, I shared the teacher's concern. She responded, "I know

*Mrs. Leeds wants me to sit still. I want to sit still.
Every day, I tell my tushie to stay in my spot in the
circle, but it doesn't listen to me."*

～～～

In the long run, Jan was very lucky that she couldn't sit
still. Despite the fact that she was smart enough to mask her
other AD/HD symptoms, her hyperactivity allowed her to
come to her teacher's attention and to eventually be diagnosed. As we will soon see, the girls with AD/HD who don't
manifest hyperactivity usually are not so lucky.

～～～

*In a typical scenario, Debbie raced two boys to the
school bus, and pushed through the line to make sure
she won the race. As she moved toward the back of
the bus, she felt someone kick her. Debbie felt pain,
anger, and humiliation. Only able to focus on her own
reactions, she lashed out without having the time to
think. Debbie never considered that perhaps this was
an accidental incident on the chaotic and overcrowded
bus. She gave no thought to the probability that her
punch would be seen by the bus driver and reported.
She had no thought that there could be a non-aggres-
sive solution to the problem, and was oblivious to the
likelihood that her peers would reject her because of
her aggressive response. Although Debbie punched
the boy she believed to be the culprit, she was still
angry as she got off the bus. On her way off, she
impulsively banged her backpack into several other
children, loudly announcing that everyone on the bus
was "a bunch of losers."   Later, the boy's mother
called Debbie's mother to discuss the incident. When*

her mother brought it up, Debbie, who was no longer angry, felt guilty and burst into tears.

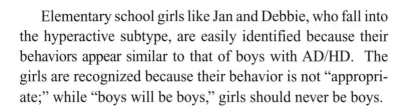

Elementary school girls like Jan and Debbie, who fall into the hyperactive subtype, are easily identified because their behaviors appear similar to that of boys with AD/HD. The girls are recognized because their behavior is not "appropriate;" while "boys will be boys," girls should never be boys.

The combined subtype

For other girls, the "hyper" quality takes on more gender-role acceptability.

A typical scenario:

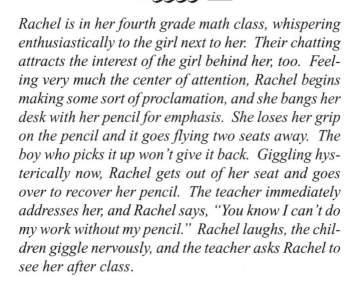

Rachel is in her fourth grade math class, whispering enthusiastically to the girl next to her. Their chatting attracts the interest of the girl behind her, too. Feeling very much the center of attention, Rachel begins making some sort of proclamation, and she bangs her desk with her pencil for emphasis. She loses her grip on the pencil and it goes flying two seats away. The boy who picks it up won't give it back. Giggling hysterically now, Rachel gets out of her seat and goes over to recover her pencil. The teacher immediately addresses her, and Rachel says, "You know I can't do my work without my pencil." Rachel laughs, the children giggle nervously, and the teacher asks Rachel to see her after class.

Rachel's behavior, while disruptive and impulsive, is not angry or aggressive. The Rachels of this world may be seen by adults as "silly," with "chutzpah," or "too busy socializing." Regardless of the interpretation, their intellect is likely to be underrated.

Primarily inattentive type

These girls bring much less notice to themselves in the classroom. They may daydream while appearing to listen to the teacher. They typically have difficulty in following directions, difficulty completing classroom assignments, and are typically messy and disorganized. At the same time, these girls are often described as sweet and shy. The confusion, frustration, and low self-esteem of these girls are internalized, as is their pain.

These are the girls who cry quietly into their pillows, and who insist to their parents that nothing is wrong. Yet, the longer the diagnosis of AD/HD is delayed, the more the symptoms of psychological stress increase. In elementary school girls, their secondary symptoms usually don't reach the level of a true disorder. Still, the tendency toward depression, anxiety or defiance is becoming clear, and should be monitored carefully. A young girl with AD/HD who says she's sorry she was born, or that there's nothing worth living for, should be taken seriously. Some parents assume that these comments are simply dramatic or manipulative, misunderstanding the intensity of emotion in their daughter. These intense feelings of unhappiness, combined with the impulsivity of AD/HD make even mild suicidal thoughts of great concern and a red flag for immediate evaluation by a professional.

Obstacles to identification

It is the super-smart girl with predominantly inattentive type of AD/HD who is least likely to be diagnosed in a timely manner. The smarter she is, the more easily she can coast through the elementary years without exhibiting overt symptoms. The smarter she is, the more easily she can compensate for her difficulties, and the more easily a teacher is willing to ignore some odd or shy behaviors. The smarter she is, the more easily her grades convince people that "there's nothing wrong." More perceptive and aware, she knows intuitively that something is very different about her, and that she's the only one who can see it. And, the more she succeeds, the more pressure there is for her to continue seeming "smart."

In these years of uneven development, high functioning girls with AD/HD will find ways of compensating. Because their symptoms are, for the most part, invisible, they may be able to mask their chronic difficulties with disorganization, lateness, and forgetfulness in school. The report cards of these smart and inattentive girls will assure their parents that their daughters are sweet, quiet, bright, but perhaps not working up to their potential. It is only at home that they can let down their defenses and be seen for the daydreamers they are.

Coping with school

There are many aspects of the elementary school situation that may be easier for the girl with AD/HD if they are handled in alternative ways.

Reading aloud for focus. When reading assignments, many girls with AD/HD find that they have the best comprehension if they read aloud to themselves. In fact, as previously discussed, Vygotsky (1978) explains that many children find this kind of "private speech" comforting, organizing, and easier to focus on than listening or reading silently. While it is a technique that works well for many girls with AD/HD, it is not acceptable in most classrooms.

Reducing distractions in the classroom. Teachers can make modifications simply by allowing these girls to sit in the front of the class, where fewer visual distractions enter their line of sight, and where they have the greatest chance of maintaining unbroken eye contact with the teacher. Surrounding the girl with AD/HD with appropriate, low-stimulation role models will also increase her chances of success.

Helping her regain focus. Touching her lightly on the shoulder when she has drifted into a daydream is a discreet way of regaining her attention while supporting her self-esteem in front of her classmates. More than being challenged by the schoolwork itself, the girl with AD/HD easily can get mired in the nuances of the school setting

Hyper-focusing in order to cope

Parents and teachers alike need to learn to recognize the possible underlying problems for girls who may appear to "try too hard" to succeed. Just as for girls in general, girls with AD/HD keenly feel the societal pressure to be neat, organized, and well-behaved (Grossman & Grossman, 1994). One common way of managing their difficulties is to develop obsessive defenses that will help them hyper-focus in order to get their work done. The ultimate achievement is not without its costs, as success involves significant struggle.

It's Sunday night at 9:00 PM. Valerie, a third grader, has just remembered that she had to make a sign for the front of her diorama, which is due tomorrow.

Valerie's mother has already told her it's bedtime and Valerie says she'll be done "in a minute." She cuts out a rectangle from a blue sheet of paper, which has a school announcement to parents on the other side. She alternately trims one side and then another until it is much smaller than she had planned. She impulsively rushes to print the words so large so that the last two letters don't fit on the sign. Frustrated, she erases furiously, wrinkling the paper, and rewrites the letters, pressing so hard that the pencil point breaks. Now, with a newly sharpened pencil, she retraces the new letters until the paper tears through in one spot. Suddenly aware that she is very tired, she chastises herself for doing such a lousy job that she has to start all over. Her mother comes in, annoyed that Valerie is still up. Valerie is ashamed to show her mother the ruined sign, and just tells her she's almost done. Her mother says it's too late to do any more work, and that Valerie needs to learn that there are consequences for forgetting to do her work. Valerie argues that "it's not fair," but her mother insists that Valerie get into bed. Valerie bursts into tears, and her mother is terribly conflicted about how to handle the situation.

For Valerie and others, obsessive tendencies are clearly a tradeoff; nonetheless, many girls with AD/HD feel they must force themselves to attend to every detail in response to societal expectations that females "have it all together," and be neat, as well.

Peers

Girls with AD/HD in elementary school have a difficult time making and maintaining friends. They don't know how to approach others, share or participate in a conversation that isn't about themselves.

In a first grade art class, Marnie wants to color in the sky on her picture and needs a blue marker, but they are all being used. Feeling ignored, she desperately shouts, "Who's got the blue?" When children say they are still using the blue markers, Marnie throws a tantrum. She stamps her feet and insists, "I HAVE to do the sky NOW!" She runs up to two of the children using blue markers and grabs the markers out of their hands, leaving blue lines across their palms. She grasps the markers tightly as she goes back to color the sky. Her classmates complain, and the teacher approaches, but Marnie does not give up the markers without a fight.

She explains to the teacher, "I needed the blue more than they did." Neediness or her desperate need to feel in control may indeed underlie Marnie's behavior. However, children and adults are likely to misinterpret this behavior. Because she is compelled to act impulsively on the primacy of her feelings, young girls with AD/HD like Marnie are often described as "rude," "bossy," "selfish," or "mean." When the teacher explains why Marnie's behavior was unacceptable, Marnie cries and says she understands. Marnie then joins her class at lunch, and gives each of the injured parties half of her lunch money. Nonetheless, the tendency to act on her impulses makes it difficult for peers to like Marnie.

The ambush

Even more confusing and frustrating for the girl with

AD/HD is the fact that when her needs overwhelm her, not even she can account for her inappropriate behavior. Such an ambush occurred while a third-grade class was rehearsing for the spring sing-along.

Melissa may have noted, for a fleeting moment, that Cathy had bumped into her twice. Because she was trying to concentrate on singing, which she loved, and on keeping her balance on the bleachers, Melissa wasn't aware of her growing annoyance with Cathy. When Louis stumbled on the bleachers and knocked into Melissa, Melissa assumed it was Cathy "bugging" her again. Too enraged to reflect, Melissa shoved Cathy off the end of the bleachers. Cathy cried, the singing stopped, and Melissa was as shocked as anyone else. Her teacher asked why she had pushed her friend. Melissa answered honestly, "I don't know." This response annoyed the teacher and Melissa was sent to the principal's office, where she cried inconsolably. Because Melissa and Cathy often had play dates together, Melissa's mother was at a loss when the principal called to report the incident. Lately, Melissa's mother had begun to dread when the phone rang after school; it seemed that often a parent or teacher was calling to complain about Melissa's behavior.

This classic experience of being ambushed—by her own reactions or by the reactions of someone else—is central to the sense of feeling "out-of-control." That being the case, it is easy to understand why so many AD/HD girls withdraw from interactions, rather than experience this loss of connectedness. These examples illustrate some of the difficulties inherent in self-monitoring with consistency—one of the critical developmental tasks that may be delayed in the girl with AD/HD.

Elementary school girls
An AD/HD-friendly user's guide
Importance of structure and routines

There are many concrete environmental changes that can be made to help a girl with AD/HD play to her strengths. The overarching goal is to create greater structure at home. This can be accomplished by instituting overt and predictable routines throughout the day, including the weekends. While these girls may say they want to be left alone to do what they desire, an outline of expectations will actually contribute to increased focus. The greatest success will be achieved if the routines are arrived at jointly with your daughter; she will feel empowered by her opportunity for input. For example, you can say, "We eat dinner at 6:00 PM every day. Do you want to take your bath before or after dinner?"

It is appropriate to expect most girls of this age to have some home responsibilities or chores. Often, a chart cataloguing these jobs can help keep her on track, and can be very useful when used in collaboration with a reward system. It can be helpful if chores are done at a routine time, daily, when a parent is present to remind and supervise. She will be able to take ownership of her responsibilities, as well as take pride in her accomplishments.

Create a realistic and predictable bedtime routine that includes reading time, brushing teeth, picking out clothes for the next school day, and whatever else you deem nonnegotiable. With consistent adherence to the routines you have created, she will gradually internalize the systems you have put in place, and feel more secure with explicit boundaries.

Time to regroup

After these girls have expended so much psychic energy holding themselves in check throughout the school day, they need a break from the task of controlling their impulses. Many girls desire play dates after school without realizing that they no longer have the energy to tolerate more intense interactions at this time. In fact, without some downtime, many play dates turn into overstimulating disasters of demands and complaints. A successful approach is to establish a "cooling off time" after school, where they can engage in more passive activities, such as watching TV, playing Nintendo, or listening to music.

It may be best not to ask her about her day at this time, but rather to wait until dinner. This period of time should belong to her, allowing her to regroup her forces and to adjust to the transition of being at home. When she does have a playdate, it should be for a short and circumscribed amount of time, with a pre-arranged activity that creates predictable expectations for both children.

Exercise—a critical tool

Exercise is an excellent outlet for all girls with AD/HD. Exercise helps channel their restless energy, and provides a physical challenge that increases focus. A healthy level of activity can shorten the time it takes them to fall asleep at night, and can improve the quality of their sleep. In addition, the endorphins released by the brain during aerobic exercise can elevate mood, just at the time of day when irritability may set in. After school is a good time to schedule exercise, whether it is bicycle riding, or a martial arts class. It is important not to overload them with activities and stimulation after school, but exercise can help release the tensions of the day, better preparing then to focus on homework later.

Keep a positive focus

Above all, it is important to treasure the creativity, spontaneity, and energy that come together to create for unique ideas and outlook. Make it clear that you are available to talk, but tolerate the fact that communication will flow most freely on her own terms. Remind her (and yourself) that you are both on the same side, and keep your sense of humor. Elementary school issues are just the tip of the iceberg; these girls will be moving into middle school, where the greater sophistication of insight and cognition combines with the wild cards of puberty and sexuality to create complex problems without easy solutions. Developing structure, self-esteem and good communication in elementary school will help these girls and their families to prepare to enter the high risk/high stress zone of middle school.

Recommendations for the parents of elementary school girls with AD/HD

- Identify and nurture her "islands of competence"—encourage her unique gifts.
- Schedule "special time," a struggle-free parent-child sanctuary that can reinforce bonding.
- Help her to develop a reminder system to avoid last minute crises; transfer as much responsibility to her as is realistic.
- Help her to learn keyboarding skills which may ease the challenge of writing assignments—a great summer activity.
- Help her to develop structured homework habits with skill repetition.
- A positive relationship with a tutor can increase confidence and competence.

QUESTIONS TO ASK YOURSELF ABOUT YOUR ELEMENTARY SCHOOL DAUGHTER

This list is designed to aid parents who may wonder about the possibility of AD/HD in their young daughters. We ask you to consider your daughter with these questions in mind. Keep in mind that some primarily inattentive girls may hide their symptoms at this age, but may exhibit more obvious signs of AD/HD when they are older. It is also important to understand that the development of different abilities progresses unevenly during the elementary school years, and that some concerning behaviors may disappear with time. Even if you answer "yes" to many of the following questions, it does not necessarily indicate the your daughter has AD/HD. However, if your concern is aroused, it may be advisable to seek the advice of a professional.

☐ Does she daydream frequently?

☐ Does she have trouble getting started on her homework?

☐ Is she easily distracted from mundane activities?

☐ Does she have trouble remembering multi-step instructions?

☐ Does she seem resistant to reading for pleasure?

☐ Does she seem oversensitive and easily embarrassed?

☐ Is she generally disorganized?

☐ Is it a struggle to get her up in the morning?

☐ Does she often have a physical complaint, such as a headache or stomachache?

☐ Is she often late for school or other activities?

- [ ] Does she "march to the beat of a different drummer?"
- [ ] Does she usually stay up past her bedtime?
- [ ] Does she often lose or misplace items?
- [ ] Does she stay at the fringe of a large group activity?
- [ ] Does she sometimes wait until the last minute to go to the bathroom?
- [ ] Does she wish she had more friends?
- [ ] Does she often lose track of the time?
- [ ] Does she tend to be shy with other children?
- [ ] Does she seem forgetful or absent-minded?
- [ ] Does she leave a trail of belongings throughout the house?
- [ ] Does she have a low frustration tolerance?
- [ ] Does she tend to interrupt conversations?
- [ ] Does she prefer to play with younger children?
- [ ] Does her teacher say she should "Speak up in class" and "Try harder"?
- [ ] Does she quickly become annoyed or irritable?
- [ ] Does she seem to overreact?
- [ ] Does she tend to put things off until later?
- [ ] Does she often seem as if she's not listening when you speak to her?
- [ ] Does she tend to blame others rather than accept responsibility?
- [ ] Is she thrown off by transitions?

- ☐ Is she often defiant and argumentative?
- ☐ Is she accident prone?
- ☐ Is she a very active "tomboy"?
- ☐ Is she a non-stop talker?
- ☐ Does she frequently interrupt?
- ☐ Does she have temper tantrums?

Chapter Seven

The Middle School Years

W hen your daughter with AD/HD reaches middle school, it is comforting to know that she has development working on her side. In other words, as she matures, she will have increasingly sophisticated cognitive abilities available to help her override her impulses. If she has been hyperactive, she will become less overtly so, especially on the gross-motor scale. Some of her symptoms will likely become less conspicuous and unwieldy, and thus more socially acceptable (which is not to say that the symptoms become milder, less pervasive, or less intrusive). Some of the long-overdue developmental steps discussed in the last chapter, such as self-monitoring, delaying need gratification, transitioning, and generalizing, are achieved during this period.

However, it is likely that your middle school daughter will

continue to lag behind her peers in terms of social skills, and that she will have a harder time academically. Middle school is a time when the core symptoms of AD/HD interfere with her abilities to meet the growing demands for independence, organization and planning, the challenges of heavier work loads, and the complex social challenges of middle school. It is a time when, due to vulnerable self-esteem and hormonal fluctuations, girls are at greater risk for psychological distress than are boys. Further, girls with AD/HD are at greater risk for psychological problems than are girls without AD/HD. Unchecked and lacking validation, their intense and mercurial emotions spark confusion and conflict that can become problematic. This distress can exacerbate AD/HD symptoms and make the disorder more complex to treat. Above all, middle-school girls have a desperate need to belong, to not be different than their peers. Regardless of the degree to which they may be suffering, it may be even more important for them to reject the idea of anything that might be viewed as a "disability." Thus, girls who were diagnosed with AD/HD in elementary school may begin to reject accommodations at school, medication, or therapy. And, girls who are referred for evaluation in middle school may fiercely reject the notion of AD/HD, claiming that they are "fine" and couldn't possibly have AD/HD like those "hyper" boys.

Developmental expectations

Erik Erikson was one of many theorists who believed that establishing one's personal identity is the central task of adolescence (Erikson, 1963). The early stages of this identity development involve gaining an understanding of one's self, one's relationship with others, and one's values and roles within society. Another task is working toward deeper and more complex relationships with peers, usually beginning with same-gender peers. Still another aspect of middle school development is a move toward more autonomy with respect to the larger world. The process of finding a balance between becoming a separate individual while remaining connected to others is one of the greatest challenges of this time period, and will continue through adolescence. It is also one of the areas where significant gender differences prevail.

Denying her own needs and feelings

Carol Gilligan has explained that girls approaching adolescence often disavow their feelings and suppress their experience—all in the name of preserving relationships (Mikel Brown & Gilligan, 1992) While all children try to live in connection to others, a girl's definition of connection involves more intimacy and more commitment than it does for a boy. In fact, a girl is willing to sacrifice to maintain those connections, even to the point of abandoning her own "voice" in order to conform to cultural gender-role expectations. While responsive relationships are essential for healthy psychological development, girls may silence themselves in relationships, rather than risk open conflict that might lead to isolation and rejection.

Indeed, psychological crises in girls' lives stem from disconnections, whether it is the beginning of normative separations from their parents, or taking the risk of asserting their "true self" before a jury of their peers. From early middle school's isolated single-sex cliques, they progress to cliques of girls interacting with cliques of boys. This is the peak period of conformity to peer behaviors and beliefs. Boys begin to see themselves as autonomous beings, able to move about freely and do as they please. On the other hand, girls decline many opportunities saying, "I can't, because my (friend, mother, sister) will feel really bad if I (do it without her, go out for that long)." In other words, for middle-school girls, there is virtually no free will without taking into account the needs of others.

Subtle encouragement to be non-assertive

Many mothers offer their daughters less encouragement to strive for independence than they do to their sons (Pipher, 1994). Rather than pushing for competence, mothers may teach their daughters about "the need not to know." In the 90's version of "smart girls should act dumb," even the brightest girls may be given the message that they should resist taking in information that will make them competent problem-solvers and forces to be reckoned with.

Instead, girls maintain "holes" in their knowledge of the world, which leads them to defer to others, whom they believe know more than they do. The "need not to know" limits them, creates dependence on others who are more knowledgeable, and ultimately serves to silence them. Mothers may lead their daughters in this direction in order for them to be accepted as an unthreatening and compliant partner. Another possibility is that they may want their daughter to remain dependent and child-like, to maintain a strong maternal connection. For girls with AD/HD, who are already mired in confusion and self-doubt, these subtle messages render them more likely to remain passive than to actively advocate for their own needs.

Puberty

Needless to say, puberty throws a monkey wrench into the works. Just as she was developing an arsenal of coping techniques that were working for her, hormonal changes create unpredictable emotional volatility and mood swings. In contrast to boys, whose hyperactivity may be abating, girl's AD/HD symptoms increase in response to the hormonal changes of puberty (Huessy, 1990). Accompanying the physical changes, impulse-driven sexual feelings are awakening and create tremendous internal confusion and distraction. These effects were discussed in depth in Chapter Four.

Lags in emotional maturity continue

Emotional maturity lags behind physical maturity in general. And, as described earlier, the emotional maturity of girls with AD/HD lags behind that of girls without AD/HD. Girls with AD/HD, who probably perceive themselves as socially awkward already, now have to contend with the novelty of bras, remembering to use deodorant, and towering over boys, whose physical maturity lags far behind that of girls. Parents may find themselves in a worrisome situation as their very immature, impulsive daughter with AD/HD develops alluring curves and starts showing an interest in boys.

Hyperactivity decreases and changes

Hyperactivity, if present earlier, begins to subside at this time. The unchanneled over-activity of childhood transforms into fine-motor fidgeting including hair twirling or chewing, cuticle picking, nail biting, and frequent doodling. Often, there is also a sense of internal restlessness. As hyperactivity decreases, other puberty-related manifestations of AD/HD take center stage, such as difficulty with peers and mood swings.

Wide swings in level of maturity

A common stance taken by girls with AD/HD at this age is one of self-righteousness, using notable phrases such as, "it's not fair" and "you don't understand"; this position often serves to alienate parents, siblings, and peers. She may respond with frustration, sarcasm and anger, as she resists anything resembling parental control. One mother described her daughter Pam in this way: "She starts to cry over something so minor, and soon it turns into hysterical sobbing. Later, she says, 'You know, Mom, I'm not a kid anymore.'" Teetering on the boundary between childhood and young womanhood, her body tells her she is no longer a kid, but her behavior often betrays her. Other AD/HD girls deny the bodily changes for as long as they can in an attempt to maintain the status quo that has provided them with security.

Diagnostic complications

It is understandable that clinicians might miss the diagnosis of AD/HD, primarily inattentive type, in a middle-school girl. The tendency of girls to internalize their symptoms makes diagnosis a challenge. Thus, the need for self-report questionnaires, such as the one offered at the end of Chapter Four.

Coexisting mood disorders and anxiety

Experts in the field of AD/HD have presented evidence indicating that the majority of persons with AD/HD also have at least one and sometimes more than one psychological or psychiatric condition (Biederman, Newcorn, & Sprich, 1991). These disorders include depression, behaviors problems, substance abuse, obsessive-compulsive disorder, anxiety disorder, and learning disabilities. More importantly, gender adds another level of complexity. At present, a review of studies seems to indicate that boys with AD/HD more commonly develop conduct and antisocial behavior disorders, while girls appear at greater risk for depression, anxiety, learning disabilities and cognitive disorders, in addition to their AD/HD diagnosis (Gaub & Carlson, 1997).

Despite all of the attention paid to the broad issues of coexisting conditions and gender, the interconnection of these two elements poses additional problems for both the diagnosis and treatment of girls with AD/HD. Indeed, when looking at girls, clinicians frequently see only the depressive symptomatology, while AD/HD often is overlooked or misdiagnosed as depression. The presence of these coexisting disorders is not disputed, but it is important to look for other possible causes for these symptoms. Could an additional source of sadness seen in these girls be the result of the guilt and shame they feel in not measuring up to society's expectations? Could it be the cognitive impairments and language difficulties associated with AD/HD, rather than learning disabilities that are the cause of academic underachievement? Could depression be the end result of this continued academic failure rather than the cause? Could poor self-esteem and depressed mood be mistaken for major depression? Is it possible that the hyperarousal of AD/HD combined with depressed mood might be misdiagnosed as bipolar illness?

It appears that children with the primarily inattentive type of AD/HD, in general, have a more significant association with anxiety disorders than do children with hyperactive/impulsive AD/HD. Anxiety may be seen in as many as 25% in this population (Biederman, J., Newcorn, J., Sprich, S., 1991). This condition has not been reported to be specifically gender-related, but appears to be more population specific, occurring most often in the AD/HD without hyperactivity group. There are, however, other conditions that appear specific to girls and under the influence of hormonal fluctuations. It is important for parents and physicians to be aware that girls with both AD/HD and anxiety may react badly to stimulant medication, which may increase her anxiety, if the anxiety is not treated concurrently. An ill-informed physician may, incorrectly, assume that a poor response to stimulants rules out an AD/HD diagnosis.

Confusion of AD/HD with depression

Many of the inattentive symptoms of AD/HD, including low energy, low self-esteem, difficulty concentrating, social withdrawal, tearfulness, and increased desire for sleep, can also be manifestations of depression. A clinician might observe classic AD/HD signs of disorganization and carelessness and construe them to be reflections of a girl feeling unmotivated due to a masked depression. Tearfulness in the office could be construed as a sign of deep hopelessness, rather than the intense and extreme emotional response that girls with AD/HD often experience. Most importantly, middle-school girls with AD/HD usually react to their underachievement and isolation by internalizing their disappointment, rather than talking about it or acting it out. In other words, the primary symptoms of AD/HD, which are often unaddressed in girls until age 12, often do result in feelings of despair and demoralization (Biederman, Mick, & Faraone, 1998). However, in this case, these symptoms are secondary to the primary AD/HD diagnosis, and reflect the pain of being long misunderstood.

The primary issue is not one of clinical depression, but the depressive symptoms may seem primary when she is evaluated by a professional. Perhaps the symptoms are exacerbated by the parents' divorce; it may be assumed that the symptoms are a clinically-depressed response to the divorce. Rather, it may be that the circumstances surrounding the divorce may be the novel and disorienting stimuli that render her usual coping strategies less effective. Perhaps her carefully hidden sadness, that reflects years of being misunderstood, intensifies. The girl's depressive features may well require treatment, but should be treated within the context of the underlying AD/HD.

Interpreting AD/HD symptoms as anxiety

Another reason middle-school girls might be taken to see a professional is because they appear worried about school. In this case, they may likely come away with a diagnosis of anxiety. Rapid speech, irritability, motoric restlessness, avoidant behavior, ruminating or obsessing, exaggerated fears, difficulty sleeping, and episodes of panic can all be presentations both of anxiety and AD/HD. However, anxiety also is a reasonable response to the relentless job of trying to compensate for AD/HD difficulties. While anxiety may seem appropriate enough in the face of the overall increase in demands on the middle-school girl, if it is impairing her daily functioning, it should be treated in the context of comprehensive AD/HD treatment.

If the anxiety experienced is secondary to the AD/HD, and not a separate co-existing disorder, it is possible that the secondary anxiety may resolve itself as the AD/HD is treated. Otherwise, the anxiety can be treated concurrent with the AD/HD treatment.

Late developing problems with school performance

The bright girl with AD/HD was probably able to coast through elementary school, compensating for her AD/HD symptoms with relatively little effort, belying the diagnostic rule-of-thumb that academic problems should be evident in early childhood (Brown, 1996). The teaching style in the elementary grades emphasizes visual materials as well as hands-on experiences, which play to the strengths of most girls with AD/HD. While she may have felt awkward inside, academic challenges were probably not experienced as particularly demanding and her achievement was generally impressive.

Often, it is in middle school that these high IQ girls begin to falter. Underachievement becomes a self-perpetuating theme that often continues throughout adolescence undermining self-esteem. A more complex curriculum, multiple teachers, less overt nurturance, and multiple classrooms, requires self-direction, greater organization, efficient memory, appropriate prioritizing, and quicker transitions—all of which are a challenge for the girl with AD/HD. In addition, social interactions increase in complexity, fueled by the hormonally-based awareness of sexuality. Taken together, all of these factors contribute to a situation with a multitude of novel demands and a significant drop in the amount of externally-imposed structure and guidance.

Demands for executive functioning increase

The ability to rely on executive brain function is a critical area for complex, multi-task functioning, and it is an area where girls with AD/HD are at a disadvantage. As previously discussed, problems with executive functioning may be manifested as difficulties with completing multi-step assignments, planning ahead, anticipating consequences, prioritizing tasks, working independently, sustaining effort and motivation, recalling and retrieving information, transitioning from one subject area to another, managing time, and staying organized.

As school demands increase in complexity, regardless of innate intelligence or acquired knowledge, girls with AD/HD need more practice and effort to be able to relegate an executive function task to automatic pilot. They may complain of cognitive fatigue towards the end of the day. In light of their energy expenditures, and in the face of hours of passive listening and sitting still, many girls find the school day an exhausting exercise. Some AD/HD girls become clock-watchers, desperately waiting for the minutes to tick by, yawning uncontrollably, unable to process any more information.

Addictive behaviors

The desire to be accepted by peers is particularly intense for all middle school students. Because girls with AD/HD already perceive themselves as different from their peers, they are even more determined to achieve a sense of belonging. Fueled by this motivation, they are willing to go to great lengths to make themselves attractive to others. Girls with AD/HD may find themselves drawn to cigarettes, alcohol, and/or drugs as avenues to peer acceptance more often than boys with

AD/HD. Alarmingly, for some, these patterns begin as early as age eleven (Biederman, 1999). Compared to boys, their stronger need for connection with others may also make the pain of social rejection more compelling for girls.

- Substance use can bring them into contact with a subculture where they may feel they have a chance of belonging, based on a shared activity.

- Addictions—to substances, food, or other behaviors—are ways of self-medicating to help them focus or slow down their thoughts.

- Addictive behaviors satisfy impulses at the same time that they provide high stimulation.

- Repetitive and/or compulsive behaviors can serve as a way of creating order and structure out of the chaos.

- Substance use may relax the girl with AD/HD who is already anxious about her interpersonal skills.

- It is developmentally expected that middle schoolers will experiment with the limits of their autonomy by taking risks.

Self-medicating with food

Food is the most common mode of self-medicating behavior, and it can easily become addictive for girls with AD/HD. The popularity of self-medicating with food is due to the fact that it is widespread, socially acceptable, introduced early in life, reinforced at home and in the media, easy to access, low-cost, and legal. The foods that girls with AD/HD seem to crave include high-sugar foods, especially coupled with carbohydrates and/or chocolate.

For many children with AD/HD, the biochemical effects of eating sugar and carbohydrates may unexpectedly provide their first experience with being able to calm their own restlessness. Eating sweets introduces a higher glucose concentration into the brain. It has been shown that as sugars and carbohydrates are metabolized, the levels of serotonin and dopamine in the brain increase. To a small degree, these food substances produce effects in the brain that are similar to the function of stimulants and other medications used to treat AD/HD. It is well documented that higher levels of these neurotransmitters can calm restlessness, as well as improve impulse control, mood, feelings of satiation, sexual energy, and sleep.

Another attraction of food is that it gratifies a primary need via a high stimulation activity. When compulsive eaters snack continuously while watching TV or a movie, the food actually may help them to focus. Some say it can create a "trance-like" state that allows them to escape for awhile from the chaos of the AD/HD brain (Nadeau, 1998). Binge eaters report that the act of planning for a binge is a high-stimulation activity in and of itself; the selection and purchase of the foods, the choice of the time and the place, and the secret and forbidden nature all contribute to the sense of excitement. For many, this adrenaline rush is more compelling and immediate than the pain of the guilt and shame that inevitably follows.

Compulsive overeating or binging are not the only dysfunctional eating patterns that may co-occur with AD/HD.

Other girls with AD/HD tend to get distracted and forget about eating. Others can't sit still at the table long enough to eat. There are also those who find the social interaction involved in a meal with others so over-stimulating that they have trouble making the cognitive transition to focusing on the food. Still others are avoidant of many tastes, textures and odors.

While boys with AD/HD may also eat compulsively, the cruelest component of indulging the impulse to eat, for girls with AD/HD, is that they are simultaneously bound by the harsh and unforgiving model of female attractiveness in our culture (Pipher, 1994). Since the constant challenge to regulate responses is central to AD/HD, a preoccupation with potentially gaining weight, or actually gaining weight, produces shame, anxiety, and low self-esteem in most girls. Girls with AD/HD, then, struggle with a classic "Catch-22": food provides them with physiological as well as psychological comfort, while simultaneously undermining their self-image and fostering guilt and shame.

Shari's story is very typical of a middle-school girl with AD/HD:

Shari, an eighth grader, still hadn't received an invitation to Rebecca's party. It was Thursday already and the party was Saturday; she wouldn't be getting an invitation this late. She wasn't invited. She knew it, but was afraid to face it. She had listened attentively when the girls at school talked about what they were going to wear to the party, and she had smiled knowingly. Now she stared at herself in her dresser mirror, as if it held the answer. She couldn't understand what was wrong with her. Suddenly, her brother Matt flung the door open without knocking. Shari screamed, "Get out, or I'll kill you!" Matt ran out, slamming the door behind him. From the impact of the slammed door, the plaster flower she had painted at Karen's birthday party crashed to the floor and broke. Shari looked down and burst into tears. She didn't realize it was the day before her period as well.

When it was quiet in the hallway, she left her room and went downstairs to the kitchen. She frantically looked in the refrigerator. She felt close to tears again and there was nothing that appealed to her. Then, she looked in the pantry and saw the cookies. Shari's mom had said those cookies were to be saved for dessert tonight, when Uncle Phil came over. Shari decided she could have a few cookies and there'd be plenty left. She didn't want anyone to see her eating them, so she took them back up to her room. She turned on VH-1 and ate the first cookie in two bites. She did the same thing with the next five. Soon, she started to feel calmer and her eating slowed a little. She forgot about Uncle Phil and Mom and Matt. She forgot that she had been dieting for Rebecca's party. When the bag was empty, she felt calm and had begun to rationalize why she didn't want to go to the party anyway. It was a full five minutes before she started to feel guilty.

AD/HD and caffeine

Another common scenario begins with a Coke, which a girl with AD/HD finds will enhance her concentration. She may start to look forward to a Coke each day, which soon increases to several caffeinated drinks daily. She begins to feel that she can only concentrate effectively when she's had some caffeine. Caffeine is a stimulant to the central nervous system, and it arouses the hypoactive AD/HD brain. Because it is easy to obtain, socially-acceptable and legal, it is not surprising that it is the drug of choice for many middle-school girls who are as yet undiagnosed. While caffeine does provide increased alertness, it is at the expense of undesired side effects, such as nervousness, irritability, and sleep disturbance.

AD/HD and nicotine

In an effort to hang out with the "cool" kids after school, the girl with AD/HD may try smoking cigarettes, even though she hates the taste. Nicotine has been shown to affect the arousal system in children with AD/HD in much the same way as stimulants. Because experimentation with these substances may fall into the category of normative developmental behaviors for the middle-school years, it is easy to overlook their potential use as a means of self-medicating. Like caffeine, nicotine also arouses the under-active part of the AD/HD brain, allowing more focused thought; it is not surprising, then, that smokers with AD/HD have the hardest time quitting.

AD/HD and alcohol

Alcohol is a central nervous system depressant that does not increase concentration, but does contribute to a feeling of relaxation and well-being. In addition to easing social awkwardness, it slows down the speeding brain for awhile (Richardson, 1997). Wendy's mother, who also has AD/HD, said, "Wendy often puts her hands over her eyes and says she wishes she could block out the tornado of thoughts and feelings, even for a few minutes. We used to call it the 'Stop the world—I want to get off' break. It took a while for me to figure out that Wendy had found wine as a way of escaping from that feeling. I found a bottle in her closet. She's probably seen me doing it often enough." For these young girls with AD/HD, the forbidden aspect of alcohol creates a high risk situation which further increases its attractiveness.

AD/HD and marijuana

Like alcohol, marijuana has a forbidden aspect, along with a cult-like mystique that attracts many girls with AD/HD. They may feel that they belong to a "cool" subculture, and that sense of belonging is a very powerful motivator. Marijuana produces a high-stimulation experience; for some, it energizes, while for others, it relaxes. In either case, it allows as an extended hyper-focus on irrelevant details that serves to slow down the AD/HD brain. It can also trigger and/or intensify impulses, such as "the munchies"; it provides a justification for out-of-control eating, drinking, or acting-out behaviors.

While marijuana does not lead to the use of harder drugs, pleasing and calming experiences with marijuana may stimulate curiosity about the effects of other mind and/or mood-altering substances. The fact that these substances can be used to self-medicate the chemical imbalances in an AD/HD brain explains some of their addictive potential. It is important to remember that these girls are experiencing strong impulsive pulls and desire for immediate gratification on a visceral level. It is helpful to understand these addictive tendencies are driven by neurological and psychological forces.

Other addictive behaviors

Still other expressions of addictive behavior can be seen in excessive or compulsive spending, working out, Nintendo play, Internet use, TV watching, sexual acting out, or shop-lifting. Most of these activities alter the brain chemistry, creating more structure and organization, which will actually yield a greater sense of control. However, this is only perceived control, because the longer-term effects of addictive behaviors have negative impacts on school, self-esteem, health, relations with parents, and even finances.

It is the long-term nature of these consequences that make them so difficult for the girl with AD/HD to see. When faced with the opportunity for powerful short-term gratification, the long-term consequences are not as compelling. So, don't make the assumption that your daughter is "just a chocoholic"; chocolate addicts also may be seeking the arousal effects of caffeine and sugar. Beginning in middle school, girls with AD/HD should be considered at risk for substance abuse, eating disorders, and other addictive behaviors.

Reducing the risk of addictive behaviors

There are many things that parents can do to help their daughters to avoid or decrease these addictive behaviors. First and foremost, be aware of tendencies toward any behavior in excess. Watch for significant and/or relatively abrupt changes in weight, mode of dress, groups of friends, ways of spending free time, secretiveness, irritability, schoolwork, or sleep patterns. Work toward making your home a safe and available haven where your daughter will feel comfortable enough to discuss her concerns. If self-medicating behaviors appear with any regularity, and she is not already being treated pharmacologically for AD/HD, consider a consultation regarding a trial of stimulant medication. Treating the chemical imbalance in her brain with medication will most likely decrease the physiological need for self-medicating behaviors. Then, with therapy aimed at behavior modification, the habitual aspect of the behavior can be addressed.

Supporting the middle school girl with AD/HD

While the hunger for peer approval is normal for this age group, the intensity of that need can be modulated. If girls have a solid mother-daughter relationship in which they feel accepted and supported, they are less likely to turn to peers as their main source of self-esteem. Certainly, the mother's tight-rope act of supporting her daughter's separation and growing independence on one hand, and the desire to protect her daughter from pain, on the other hand, is one of the most bitter-sweet passages of parenthood. Speaking frankly with her about the changes in her body and her feelings lets her know that these things are normal, and not one more thing that makes her "different." Acknowledging that middle school is a confusing time, with lots of new feelings and distractions, will validate her experience. A mother also can normalize her daughter's experience. Let her know that you felt the same way when you were her age. Chances are that she may not have felt comfortable enough to discuss this with her friends, or perhaps it flies out of her mind in the face of so many stimuli at school. Above all, make sure she knows that you embrace her as she is.

Structured activities

Another way to create an AD/HD-friendly environment is to help her get involved in structured and supervised activities. Whether it is a sports activity, a community service organization, a religious youth group, or a drama group, these activities provide a built-in peer group. Adults circumscribe the activity, the time frame, and the ground rules for interactions. Usually, the inattentive types prefer activities that occur in a small intimate group; the more hyper-emotional types can play to a larger and more varied audience. And, in the event that there is the inevitable misunderstanding with a peer, there will be a good number of potential acquaintances that remain. An activity imposes another piece of routine on her life, and offers another arena for gaining self-esteem. This is especially valuable if her school performance is flagging, and doesn't provide a source of pride at this time. Finally, from a practical standpoint, involvement in sanctioned activities will offer her less time and incentive to pursue riskier avenues. Parents can reinforce the importance of these activities by showing their support, whether by participating in a carpool to get her there, being present at the team games, or volunteering to supervise or chaperone, just to name a few possibilities.

Coaching

A coach can be a helpful addition to the support network for a middle schooler with AD/HD. If the coach is following up on the girl's responsibilities, parents are freer to remove themselves from the intense power struggle that is inevitable. Most AD/HD girls are resistant to pursuing projects that are inherently uninteresting to them. While negotiating is a necessity, the role of policeman is better left to someone who does not share the emotional investment in your daughter's success. An all-too-familiar scenario was described by Terry's father:

"When I get home in the evening, I'm in charge of the homework detail. Terry argues about everything, whether or not she has homework, how much homework she has, how long it will take her to do it, what time she should start it, when she should take a break. You can't imagine the battles we have. After I haven't seen her all day, I hate for this to be the basis of our relationship, and often we are struggling up until her bedtime. We both agree that I have become more of a policeman than a dad, and neither of us likes it. I was complaining about this to Terry's psychologist and she suggested we try a coach. Since we hired Julie, my interactions with Terry are fun and loving, and she gets her work done, too. A coach is one of the best investments I've ever made."

As Carol Gilligan has described, this is the age when girls begin to lose their "voice." Parents can reinforce the value of that inner voice, and support the strength that is needed to maintain it amidst a culture that tends to silence girls. As mentioned earlier, research shows that levels of anxiety and depression increase at the end of middle school for girls with AD/HD (Huessy, 1990). As these girls make the transition into adolescence, they struggle to plant their feet firmly beneath them. Whether they lurch in all directions at once, or pull back into a turtle shell, no one can protect them from being buffeted about by unpredictable winds. Ultimately, girls with AD/HD must learn for themselves that they cannot change the wind, but they can learn to adjust their sails.

QUESTIONS TO ASK YOURSELF ABOUT YOUR MIDDLE-SCHOOL DAUGHTER

This list is designed to aid parents who may wonder about the possibility of ADHD in their middle school daughters. We ask you to consider your daughter with these questions in mind. Even if you answer "yes" to many of the following questions, it does not necessarily indicate the your daughter has AD/HD. However, if your concern is aroused, it may be advisable to seek the advice of a professional.

☐ Does she daydream frequently?

☐ Does she have trouble getting started on her homework?

☐ Is she easily distracted from mundane activities?

☐ Does she forget things she's supposed to do?

☐ Does she seem resistant to reading for pleasure?

☐ Does she seem oversensitive and easily embarrassed?

☐ Is she generally disorganized?

☐ Is it a struggle to get her up in the morning?

☐ Does she often have a physical complaint, such as a headache or stomachache?

☐ Is she often late for school or other activities?

☐ Does she "march to the beat of a different drummer?"

☐ Does she usually stay up later at night than you'd like?

☐ Does she often lose or misplace items?

☐ Does she stay at the fringe of a large group activity?

☐ Does she wish she had more friends?

☐ Does she often lose track of the time?

☐ Does she tend to be shy with her peers?

☐ Does she seem forgetful or absent-minded?

☐ Does she leave a trail of belongings throughout the house?

☐ Does she have a low frustration tolerance?

☐ Does she tend to interrupt conversations?

☐ Does she seem immature for her age?

☐ Does her teacher say she should "Speak up in class" or "Try harder?"

☐ Does she quickly become annoyed or irritable?

☐ Does she seem to overreact?

☐ Does she tend to put things off until later?

☐ Does she often seem like she's not listening when you speak to her?

☐ Does she tend to blame others rather than accept responsibility?

☐ Is she thrown off by transitions?

Chapter Eight

The High School Years

The high school years are often a difficult and challenging time. It seems as if nature and society have conspired to pack these four years with so many daunting challenges that even the most adept and well-adjusted adolescent feels overloaded. When AD/HD is added to the mix, high school becomes more challenging, and may even become a destructive experience. In this chapter, we examine the particular vulnerabilities for girls with AD/HD in high school and suggest ways that parents, teachers, and other professionals can offer much-needed support.

Issues of late diagnosis for teenage girls

Because girls behave very differently, because they work harder to hide their academic difficulties and to conform to teacher expectation, because they are often misdiagnosed as anxious and/or depressed in adolescence and young adulthood, late diagnosis is very common in girls with AD/HD. Girls who are particularly bright often are able to compensate for their AD/HD much longer, and are therefore the most likely candidates for a late diagnosis.

Awareness and advocacy for girls diagnosed late

Parents and professionals alike need to be aware of the reasons for late diagnosis and to consider the possibility of AD/HD when a girl starts to experience academic difficulties in high school, or even later during college. The fact that her AD/HD symptoms may not have been apparent in early years renders her AD/HD no less real when it rears its head in adolescence, a time when the demands for planning, organization, recall, and focus intensify. Unfortunately, skepticism is common on the part of educators when a late diagnosis occurs. Girls who are diagnosed late may need extra support and advocacy from parents and professionals as they may encounter resistance when they request accommodations on standardized testing for college entrance, or as they need other accommodations and support in their high school years.

Issues for adolescent girls with AD/HD

Social pressures

Social deficits, present in earlier years, often have their greatest impact during adolescence as girls begin to separate from family and move into the all-important social milieu of high school. During the high school years, girls begin to move out of the all-girl cliques of middle school and begin to explore their individuality in both same sex and opposite sex relationships. The more complex high school social patterns often call for a level of awareness and self-control that many girls with AD/HD don't possess. Their social deficits result in the sad, but common tale told by women with AD/HD—that they were never quite able to navigate successfully in their social milieu during adolescence.

Social pressures are intense for all students during adolescence, with enormous energy expended on peer analysis: watching, imitating, relating, comparing, and conforming. In addition to this exhausting list, girls with AD/HD often feel despair. The phrases we hear repeated again and again by women with AD/HD, recalling their adolescent years, are "I didn't fit in," or "I always felt different, but I never knew why." Many report having "no friends" or "only one best friend," while others recall their adolescent years as a blur of impulsive behavior, promiscuity, and heavy drinking in a desperate effort to gain acceptance. Those who did manage to succeed academically often had no time at all for social life, paying an extra high price for top grades.

"In high school I was shy and really didn't have any friends. I just felt like I never fit in with any type of people. I didn't feel I was smart, but I never wanted to hang out with the 'rough crowd' either."

Family support and acceptance is critical, but can never entirely counteract the damage that can be done to teenagers who feel rejected by their peer group. The very negative self-image that girls with AD/HD may develop during high school can haunt them for years afterwards.

Gender expectations conflict with AD/HD traits

If we examine some of the pressures and expectations often placed on teenage girls, it is easy to see how they can come into direct conflict with AD/HD traits or tendencies. For example, girls are typically encouraged to be neat, "feminine" (controlled and passive), carefully groomed (in order to be attractive to the opposite sex), sensitive to the feelings of others, and compliant toward adults.

A teenage girl with AD/HD may respond anxiously, even obsessively, to the expectation that she be well groomed and fashionably dressed. She may be unable to organize her room or her life well enough to have clean, color-coordinated clothing available on a given school morning. This may lead to frantic, screaming tirades as she searches through piles of clothing on the floor, the dirty clothes basket, or her sister's closet. She may impulsively grab something to wear at the last minute, as she races out the door for school—very likely leaving behind some crucial item in her rush.

The self-doubts and competitiveness so common among teenage girls are often more intense for girls with AD/HD, and hurt feelings can escalate more rapidly into impulsive remarks or over-reactions. Once the drama is over, she may be ready to forgive and forget. Yet a girl with AD/HD often finds herself facing rejection by her peers who are stung by her comments and become intolerant of her outbursts.

Of course, there is overlap between the dilemmas of teenage boys with AD/HD and teenage girls with AD/HD. Girls aren't the only ones who may feel socially excluded. But girls seem to feel much more intense reactions to social difficulties than do boys with AD/HD during adolescence. This may, in part, be due to the fact that AD/HD-like behaviors, such as risk-taking, arguing, defiance, and being action-oriented, are more socially acceptable for boys. Similar traits in girls, however, can be met with criticism, and even ostracism.

Boys may engage in group activities or group sports without being required to exhibit the same level of social skills that are expected from a girl. Interrupting, contradicting, or reacting angrily when frustrated will only result in social ostracism among boys if they occur repeatedly in the extreme. Boys can retreat behind athletics, computers, or even behind a "who cares" attitude if social skills are lacking.

The struggle to "measure up"

Many women with AD/HD report that they were able to find and keep friends more successfully after their adolescent years were behind them. Fortunately, in college and beyond, they find a more varied range of choices in their quest for a social niche. Once they are among more mature and tolerant people who don't demand such a high degree of conformity, they are able to more readily find relationships. However, they will likely find throughout their lives that their feelings of differentness and lack of acceptance re-emerge whenever they encounter women who are highly competitive, judgmental, or who highly value self-control or orderliness. The goal in helping these girls during adolescence is for them to learn to value themselves, and to seek the company of people who can appreciate their strengths. Through building awareness of their strengths and special gifts, they can avoid falling into a pattern of self-reproach for their inability to "measure up" to the standards of social convention.

Pressures to "mature"

Pressure to grow up and become responsible increase during adolescence. Sometimes parental expectations for their daughters to demonstrate "maturity" can come into direct conflict with the neuro-cognitive patterns associated with AD/HD. This doesn't mean that our daughters can't become "mature," but it does mean that maturity needs to be viewed through an AD/HD lens. In other words, it is important to recognize those areas that pose a much greater challenge for girls with AD/HD. What we call "maturity" typically involves the ability to make and follow plans, to postpone immediate gratification, to consider consequences, to moderate emotional reactions, to reliably do what we've been asked to do, to learn from the past, and to plan for the future. Many of these signs of "maturity" are capacities related to the functions of the frontal lobes of the brain, and it is the frontal lobes that are primarily affected by AD/HD.

What does this mean to the adolescent girl with AD/HD? She may be more forgetful, less reliable, and have much more difficulty in planning and carrying out long term assignments. In general, she may be more prone to feeling overwhelmed by the multiple demands of school, extracurricular activities, social life, and part-time work. The hopeful news, however, is that frontal lobes continue to develop throughout adolescence and young adulthood, increasing her ability to effectively take charge of her life.

High school and AD/HD—not a good "fit"

Pressures and demands seem to reach a crescendo in high school because there is so little choice and flexibility. High school is designed in a way that seems almost diabolically structured to be AD/HD-unfriendly. The day starts too early and lasts too long—with demands for focus and concentration that far exceed the capacity of most students, even those without AD/HD. There is little choice in the array of courses required for graduation. Many students with AD/HD are placed in the position of being forced to read about and study subjects that hold little or no interest for them—something they should be strongly advised against doing once they are graduated from high school! And yet, during the high-school years, they don't have many options to customize their courses and activities. (In Chapter Nine, the reader will find much more detailed information about *how* to deal with the AD/HD-unfriendly high school years).

Once high school is behind her, the teenage girl with AD/HD will have more choices open to her: she can work full-time, go to school full-time, or do a combination of the two. She will have many different types of jobs and academic settings from which to choose, and can actively avoid placing herself in a situation where she is required to concentrate for long periods on topics of little interest.

Conformity and compliance

Many forces are at work for both boys and girls with AD/HD, making it difficult for them to excel in high school. However, there is added pressure for girls because of their greater needs for social acceptance, for meeting the expectations of parents and teachers, as well as their overall greater desire to conform. Girls with AD/HD may be more prone to anxiety —an outgrowth of this desire to please, to do what is expected. Their efforts to compensate in order to meet expectations may mask their AD/HD struggles, making their difficulties more likely to be overlooked by parents and teachers. As it becomes increasingly challenging for them to meet expected demands, their anxiety level often rises. It is much more difficult for a girl to live with the consequences of AD/HD and still feel good about herself.

All of the social conditioning that told her as a little girl that she should be "good" (sweet, compliant, clean, and tidy) doesn't disappear, even though it may seem so. If you are a parent who has daily screaming battles with your daughter, you may read this with skepticism. What great desire to conform? All she does is argue! Although she may be very emotionally volatile and may strongly resist your attempts to control her, she still lives with an inner struggle. Your little girl who had stomach aches because she couldn't manage to do what the teacher asked, is still alive and well somewhere inside. We know this through listening to the recollections of grown women with AD/HD. Whether or not she lets you know it, it is likely that she feels deeply wounded when she is criticized by parents, teachers, and others. She may compare herself unfavorably to the successes of her peers, as well. Although as a teen she may feign indifference to negative opinions, later she will have painful recollections of this period of her life.

The emotional roller coaster

Teenage girls with AD/HD tend to be more emotionally reactive than other girls, and to have a harder time moderating their responses. Whether it is frustration over a homework assignment, distress over her appearance, anger at a younger sibling who "borrowed" her sweater, despair over feeling socially isolated, or anger at parents who "treat her like a baby," the emotional roller coaster that is adolescence tends to be more extreme for a girl with AD/HD.

It is critical that parents and professionals recognize that this intensity has a neurological basis, and that reactions tend to become even more extreme during times of stress, fatigue, hunger, or Pre-Menstrual Syndrome (PMS). Both the teenage girl and her parents need to recognize the added vulnerability that she has, and begin to identify and manage the potential stresses that can worsen her reactions.

The impact of hormones

In a short, four-year period our daughters with AD/HD move from girlhood to the brink of womanhood. Tremendous hormonal changes occur, and the hormonal fluctuations of the menstrual cycle intensify and complicate the confusion and unpredictability that are part and parcel of growing up with AD/HD. While PMS may be an annoying period of irritability, fatigue, or cramping for many girls, those with AD/HD may feel such an increase in the intensity of their emotional reactions, irritability, and low frustration tolerance, that they require active intervention. Physicians, therapists and others who treat adolescent girls with AD/HD should be aware of this added vulnerability, and take steps to keep up-to-date on research on PMS and on new approaches for minimizing its impact. The use of anti-depressant medication to combat the effects of PMS is fairly well-known, but recent research has suggested that there are a number of ways to reduce PMS symptoms in the more vulnerable AD/HD population (see Chapter 11).

Sexual risks

Teenage girls with AD/HD may be at greater risk for

pregnancy than are other teenage girls (Arnold, 1996). This may be true for a number of reasons. Teenage girls who struggle with low self-esteem, as do many girls with AD/HD, may seek affirmation through the sexual attentions of boys in an effort to compensate for feelings of inadequacy in other areas of their life. Furthermore, due to difficulties with impulse control, poor planning ability, and inconsistency, many of these girls are prone to have unprotected sex, use birth control inconsistently, and/or have multiple partners. As a result, these girls may be among the most at-risk for contracting a sexually-transmitted disease or having an unwanted pregnancy during high school. This difficult reality of unplanned pregnancies among these girls is reflected in the high percentages of children with AD/HD who are placed for adoption.

What can parents and professionals do to help reduce this risk?

- Support groups for girls with AD/HD can help them feel more accepted and less alone, reducing their need to seek male sexual attention.

- Helping them become involved in structured, constructive activities will give them other outlets to develop self-esteem. Recent studies confirm what common sense tells us: adolescents who are kept busy in extracurricular activities, sports, church groups, and so on are less likely to get in trouble during high school.

- An open, supportive relationship with their parents gives them somewhere to turn for advice if they do become sexually active—either to help them make a wise choice of birth control or to help make the best decision if they do accidentally become pregnant.

- Helping them find and develop "islands of competence" is highly beneficial. The girl who has many sources of support and self-esteem will be much less needy, and therefore less vulnerable to sexual attention.

Risks associated with driving

Studies of teens with AD/HD have shown that, in general, they have a greater likelihood of being involved in traffic accidents. One study reported that teens with AD/HD had significantly more accidents. The researchers attributed this higher accident rate to problems with attention and cognitive control (Beck et al., 1996). Most studies have only examined the driving behavior of boys with AD/HD, but one study in New Zealand (Nada-Raja et al., 1997) studied both boys and girls and found that girls with attentional difficulties were at high risk for both traffic crashes and driving offenses.

The important message for parents is that their daughters with AD/HD may need more practice in driving so that driving skills become more automatic and require less concentrated effort and attention. Secondly, since attention problems seem to be strongly implicated in traffic accidents, girls (and boys) with AD/HD should take care to drive in less distracting situations during their first years as a driver. They should avoid heavy traffic, social distractions, such as excited, talkative peers, and, it goes without saying, should never drink and drive. Teens with AD/HD must maintain a more conscious awareness of their need to "keep their eyes on the road."

In order to avoid accidents even in adulthood, individuals

with AD/HD may find themselves distracted by conversation while driving. For less experienced drivers, such a distraction could be all it takes to trigger a chain reaction leading to an accident. Thirdly, situations that may lead to impulsive reactions should be discussed in advance and avoided, if possible. Such situations might include driving with peers who are impulsive risk-takers, or who have been drinking and who may encourage a teenage girl with AD/HD to take a risk "for fun."

Risk of anxiety and depression

Parents and professionals need to be watchful during the teenage years to assess whether the "normal" emotional roller coaster for girls with AD/HD has careened over the edge into a level of anxiety or depression that requires treatment in tandem with her treatment for AD/HD. Emotions can tip quickly when environmental stresses suddenly overwhelm the teenage girl's already distressed system. An accidental pregnancy, the breakup of a relationship, a failed exam, a rejection letter from a college—any of these might be enough to push her into levels of anxiety or depression that may require both medication and psychotherapy.

"I spent a lot of lonely times in my room. I look back on it now and believe that I suffered through depression during those years. I kept it so well-hidden, that my mom and dad never knew." —Chris D.

Risk for substance abuse and addictive behaviors

We have discussed these issues in detail in the preceding

chapter on the middle school years. Such risks, of course, continue and intensify as an increasing number of peers are involved in smoking cigarettes, drinking alcohol, smoking marijuana, and experimenting with a range of other drugs. A recent study (Biederman et al., 1999) reports that 14% of girls with AD/HD have a substance use disorder, and one in five smoke cigarettes. As teens with AD/HD reach age 16 or 17 and obtain their driver's licenses, the dangers associated with drinking and drugs increase greatly. Parents who are concerned about the possibility of impulsive drinking and driving should very carefully consider whether the convenience of having a teen that can transport herself is worth the potentially lethal results of combining drugs or alcohol and driving.

Developmental issues: separating from childhood dependence upon parents

High school is a time to gradually separate from the dominance and control of parents. But this transition is often intensified and prolonged when AD/HD is in the picture. Along with the normal impulses toward independence comes a gnawing, rarely expressed fear that she can't really handle the responsibility and expectations of self-reliance that accompany her growing freedom. This combination can make the high-school years an exceptionally bumpy ride as teenage girls with AD/HD demand more independence only to feel overwhelmed, even frightened by the dilemmas created through their impulsivity, disorganization, and poor planning.

If your daughter is the quiet, daydreamy type, she may engage in less of the behavior that can be so frightening for parents—defying parental rules, drinking, experimenting with drugs, or early sexual behavior. But these years are still likely to be fraught with pain for her. Many quiet, shy young women with AD/HD report having felt too intimidated to practice the skills needed to be self-sufficient when they leave home.

Developing skills for independent living

Parents can help their daughters gain skills for autonomy and independence by remaining patient, and by recognizing that the process may take their daughter longer than the average adolescent. Advance practice can be helpful.

➤ If she hopes to go away from home to college, she may benefit greatly by attending a school that offers an extended orientation period in the summer before freshman year for students who have special needs.

➤ It may be very helpful to open a checking account during high school, where she can deposit any cash gifts or money earned from summer jobs. In this fashion, she has a longer period of time to learn the habit of recording checks and keeping an accurate account balance.

➤ Learning to handle charge cards responsibly is crucial to adult life, but can be very difficult for any teen. Obtaining a card with a very low limit—$200-$300—can provide experience without opening the door to disaster.

➤ Providing her with a clothing allowance during high school also can give her experience in managing money, setting priorities, and making decisions within defined limits.

- Learning to use a day planner is one of the most critical skills your daughter needs to master as she leaves home for college or the working world. A day planner is not only for recording appointments, but for recording all crucial information—phone numbers, addresses, shopping lists, directions, and so on. By developing the habit of writing all-important information in one place, she will have a skill that is invaluable for managing AD/HD tendencies toward forgetfulness and disorganization.

- The simple act of setting an alarm clock and depending upon oneself to get up on time in the morning is often very challenging for girls with AD/HD. This is a skill best practiced at home, where parents can remain a back-up system, rather than waiting until she is away at college, or in her first apartment.

- All students face increasing, multiple demands as they enter their high school years—multiple teachers and assignments, extra-curricular activities, part-time jobs, increased responsibilities to help at home, learning to drive, beginning to date—the list is long and daunting. Girls with AD/HD will need help in organizing and managing these multiple demands, and in making AD/HD-friendly choices so that they are not juggling more than they can manage. Working with a coach who specializes in AD/HD can often be very helpful for girls as they learn to organize and prioritize.

Learning to embrace her strengths

"I'm just not good at anything," Lisa, a ninth grade girl with AD/HD, expressed despairingly. With regret and envy she described girls in her class who had made the cheerleading squad, earned top grades, or had already completed years of music or dance lessons, developing high levels of skill and self-confidence in the process. Lisa had taken up and dropped many interests—a pattern typical for girls with AD/HD. At age 14, she no longer had faith in herself or in her capacity to stick with any endeavor. Easily discouraged, and with a low-frustration tolerance, she pursued each succeeding interest with less and less faith that she would discover a talent or develop a skill.

Girls who have developed ability or talent in some area seem to be much better inoculated against Lisa's cloud of self-defeating gloom. Teachers and parents may shrug off a girl's declaration that she has "no idea what she wants to do," reassuring her that most people don't figure that out until later. However, what they may not recognize is the particular vulnerability of girls with AD/HD, who may have very little sense of accomplishment or ability. Rather than simply not having pinpointed a career path, these girls often suffer from a belief that they possess no valuable talent or ability.

One of the most constructive approaches in helping a girl with AD/HD through her high school years is to actively help her develop and recognize areas of competence and talent. This is a first step toward helping her learn about herself and what types of post-high school training and employment would work well for her. It is important to consider not just her AD/HD, but her abilities, interests, and personality as well. These girls often have a well-developed sense of what they're *not* good at, but very little awareness of their strengths. Awareness of strengths and abilities has a far greater value than its utilitarian value in career counseling. The more that girls with AD/HD are in touch with their areas of competence, the less vulnerable they will be to the criticisms and frustrations that so often accompany AD/HD.

The most therapeutic process for girls with AD/HD is to begin to develop a sense of competence and ability. There are many arenas in which to do this, and exploration shouldn't be limited to career possibilities. Part-time work after school, even though it competes with study time, may give her a chance to feel capable, and to receive evidence of this in the form of a paycheck. Volunteering at a local hospital or nursing home, helping to build props for the school play, participating in a community beautification project, learning to ride horseback—these activities may not directly evolve into a career path, but can be enormously beneficial in helping her to build a sense of self-confidence.

Learning assertiveness and self-advocacy

Saying "no" is not typically included in the set of tools with which girls are equipped. Rather, they are taught to be cooperative, compliant, and helpful. Many girls with AD/HD try to fade into the woodwork, fearing any interaction that may call upon them to be assertive. Sari Solden (1995) writes extensively, in her book *Women with Attention Deficit Disorder,* about the difficulty that most women with AD/HD have in being appropriately assertive in expressing their needs for assistance or accommodation. Those girls whose AD/HD is more "external," like many boys, may say "no" frequently, but may not do so with diplomacy and grace. They are labeled as "having an attitude," or worse.

The difficulty of learning to advocate for needs related to AD/HD compounds the assertiveness challenge for a girl. Added to the self-consciousness and self-doubts that any teen with AD/HD might experience when they first attempt to express their needs, girls have the extra burden of having been trained, since their earliest years, to compromise, comply, and not be "bossy" or "demanding."

"I remember my mother always saying to me in elementary school and high school that I shouldn't be so difficult, so bossy. She'd tell me that I wouldn't have any friends and the teachers wouldn't like me if I didn't try harder to be 'nice'." —Cara

The high-school years are the time in which a girl needs to develop the self-advocacy skills needed for more independent life beyond high school—whether in an educational setting or in the workforce. She will need to be able to express her needs confidently and convincingly to professors or employers who are ill-informed about AD/HD. She needs validation of her right to express her opinion, and help in learning to express it in a constructive, effective manner.

High schools often stress the need for students with AD/HD to become their own self-advocates, rather than continue to rely on parents. However, few high schools provide help in learning these crucial skills! This is another area where a girls AD/HD support group can provide enormous benefit. In this kind of setting girls can practice with each other, commiserate with each other when they feel intimidated or embarrassed in their efforts, and receive counsel about the best ways to explain and assert their needs.

Coaching and benefits of structure

As with girls of all ages with AD/HD, teenage girls need support, encouragement, and structure. Because teenage girls are trying to develop more independence, sometimes it is more helpful when someone other than her parents provides structure. This could be a therapist, coach, or school guidance counselor.

Coaching can be helpful at younger ages, but as the girl with AD/HD enters her high-school years, coaching may be a key element in her efforts to learn to meet the greatly increased demands for organization and planning. It is critical for teenage girls to collaborate with their coach rather than feeling that the coach is just one more adult in her life who instructs and restricts her. Good rapport between the coach and teen is essential. Parents need to take a more backseat role, allowing their teenage daughter, together with the coach, to set the agenda. Working with a coach throughout high school can help a teenage girl with AD/HD construct a critical bridge between childhood dependence and the demands for increasing independence as she leaves home for college or independent living a few short years later.

These are the years when the teenage girl needs to take on the notion that learning to be on time, developing tools to improve her organization, setting priorities rather than staying in a reactive mode, are for her own benefit, not something imposed by parents.

College placement counseling

As the teenage girl with AD/HD approaches her junior year

of high school, she and her family should be working together very actively to make good decisions regarding what she will do after high school. The assistance of a specialized college placement counselor can be especially useful to help her and her parents sort through the maze of possibilities: community college, vocational training, attending a four-year college while remaining at home, going away to a small college, or applying to a large university. Not only are there a huge variety of educational settings to choose from, but also there is a wide range in the degree of support available for students with AD/HD at various educational institutions.

The most critical element in the decision-making process is to accurately assess her level of maturity, her readiness to leave the structure and security of home, her need for academic support, and her preferences regarding the atmosphere, geographic location, and courses of study offered by various schools. This daunting process should not be left for the teenage girl with AD/HD to address alone. However, she should be an active participant, expressing her preferences and desires, and taking part in visiting, interviewing, and considering her options.

Most teens with AD/HD need a high level of support when faced with the formidable task of writing college essays, asking for letters of recommendation, and completing application forms. Because tension often runs high between parents and teens around this process, primary support is sometimes best provided by a coach or tutor.

Career counseling/ability testing

The latest statistics still show that women, at all educational levels, earn less than men with the same level of training. Social stereotypes continue to strongly influence not only the hiring practices of employers, but also the career choices that young women pursue. Typically, many of the jobs performed by women involve caring for, supporting, or "administratively assisting" others. Often, it is just these sorts of jobs that are particularly unsuitable for women with AD/HD because they involve *being* the support system for others, rather than allowing them to *build* a support system around themselves. The very tasks of reminding, attending to details, organizing, and assisting with paperwork are the tasks that are typically the least-suited to the AD/HD brain.

"When I graduated from high school, I didn't have a clue as to what my interests or strong points were. I did end up going to a community college, taking secretarial classes. But after going there for two years, I decided that it was too boring. I was the only one in the family who didn't know what they wanted to do. I just didn't seem to have any ambition. After college, I got the idea that I wanted to be a hairdresser, so I went to a beauty school. I remember my dad saying, 'I'll pay for it as long as you get a job out of it.' I said I would. I got a job, but I hated it. I was so bad at it I quit. I couldn't keep up with the pace and I just lost interest. I really felt like a failure. To this day I don't know what kind of job would be good for me." (A 29-year-old with AD/HD who is now seeking career guidance.)

Girls in high-school need to be educated about AD/HD-friendly jobs and work environments so that their career selections and job paths are not ill-chosen. Assessment of high-school girls with AD/HD should include career interest and ability testing, as well as the Myers-Briggs Type Inventory.

Such tests can become the basis of helping them identify strengths and talents, and can be of enormous value in helping the girl with AD/HD make good choices of jobs or of courses of study in college. Without this kind of assistance and guidance, many young women with AD/HD will experience repeated failure and frustration as they move from one inappropriate career path to the next.

Conclusion

The high-school years are among the most challenging years of life for an individual with AD/HD, and especially for girls with AD/HD. To bridge the challenges of high school, they need support from peers, parents, and schools, combined with appropriate medical treatment, depending on their particular needs and issues. With the right supports and interventions, these girls can make the crucial transition from the chaos and self-doubt of adolescence to a sense of growing strength, efficacy, and competence as they enter their young adult years.

—∼∽∼—

QUESTIONS TO ASK YOURSELF ABOUT YOUR TEENAGE DAUGHTER

This list is designed to aid parents who may have questions about the possibility of AD/HD in their teenage daughter. We ask you to take a look at your daughter with these questions in mind. Some signs of AD/HD in teens can be confusing because they may be behaviors typical of all teens, but are perhaps more marked in teens with AD/HD. It may be helpful to look at the questions for parents of middle-school, elementary school and preschool aged daughters and to answer them retrospectively, looking back at your daughter's behavior at younger ages. Keep in mind, however, that many girls do not exhibit obvious signs of AD/HD in their younger years. You should not rule out the possibility of AD/HD if your daughter seems to exhibit signs now, but did not exhibit them earlier. Even though you may answer "yes" to many of the following questions, this does not necessarily indicate that your daughter has AD/HD , but if your concerns are aroused, it may be advisable to seek a professional evaluation.

☐ Does she have great difficulty in planning and organizing long-term assignments?

☐ Does she have a strong tendency to procrastinate?

☐ Does she tend to study and/or write papers at the last minute, possibly staying up all night?

☐ Does she seem flighty or scattered?

☐ Does she have trouble getting to sleep at night and waking in the morning?

☐ Does she leave a trail of belongings in every room she passes through?

☐ Does she frequently misplace keys, umbrellas, and other personal belongings?

☐ Does she seem overwhelmed by school?

☐ Is she hyper-verbal?

☐ Does she tend to interrupt frequently in conversation?

☐ Do her emotional reactions, both positive and negative, seem out of proportion to the event?

☐ Does she appear to have difficulty with anxiety or depression?

☐ Do you feel that her academic achievement is significantly below her intellectual potential?

☐ Does she need to work in a rigid, almost compulsive fashion for long hours to complete her work?

☐ Does she work hard for teachers she likes, but very little for teachers she dislikes?

☐ Does she have a pattern of starting out well during the school year, but losing steam as the year progresses?

☐ Is she often late?

☐ Is she forgetful, absentminded?

☐ Are you concerned about her judgement regarding drinking, driving and sexuality?

☐ Are you concerned about drug experimentation?

☐ Does she have low frustration tolerance?

☐ Does she frequently forget important items at home and at school?

☐ Does she seem to have an exceptionally difficult time during her PMS week?

☐ Does she smoke cigarettes?

☐ Does she drink large quantities of caffeinated drinks?

☐ Does she engage in binge eating?

☐ Does she tend to drop hobbies, interests, activities?

☐ Are habits hard for her to develop?

☐ Do her habits seem overly rigid?

☐ Does she seem stressed much of the time?

Chapter Nine

Educational Issues

O ur daughters with AD/HD will face special challenges to receive the educational supports that they need. First, few parents and teachers are informed enough to recognize the signs of AD/HD in the majority of girls who are affected. Secondly, most girls have not been trained to be assertive, and girls whose self-esteem has been damaged are even less prepared to ask for what they need. In addition, these girls create fewer dilemmas for the classroom teacher. Because they are not usually disruptive, most teachers will, quite naturally, focus on those students, more often boys, who are causing problems for the teacher and for other students. And, finally, the demand for "special education" services is of almost tidal wave proportions, greatly exceeding the supply. Girls with AD/HD are unlikely to be at the head of the line.

In this chapter, we want to emphasize a team approach to helping girls with AD/HD in school. This approach strongly encourages parents not to place the responsibility for helping their daughters entirely in the hands of the school, but rather to form a team, some members of which may be private coaches, tutors, and therapists, who, working together with parents and teachers can help her to recognize and realize her full potential.

But before we begin to outline educational approaches that can better support our daughters with AD/HD, let's listen to the voices of women who did not have the benefit of identification and support during their school years. Perhaps by hearing their accounts we can develop a clearer notion of how to respond to the needs of girls growing up today.

Sally, now in her forties, was a bright, athletic tomboy who grew up climbing trees and competing with her brothers. Although very outgoing, Sally recalls preferring the company of boys, with whom she felt more at home, to the company of her female peers, where she never quite "fit in."

"When I was in school, teachers would say that I never stopped talking. I was very social, always busy doing something, and not paying attention to my lessons. On my report cards only one teacher 'caught it' (my AD/HD) and said that I was inconsistent and made careless errors. The other teachers just patted me on the head and said I was fine.

No one expected me to be a scholar. I was told my whole life that I was 'average.' I didn't make A's and no one expected me to. I earned a strong B average with no effort. I didn't realize I was smart until I got to college, but even there I had no direction and kept changing my major every time I met a professor that I liked.

With more guidance and structure I would have been able to develop. As it was, it felt like I was slogging through a swamp—trying to get where I was going, but every step I sank down to my knees—I kept going, but I never knew where I was."

Sally's experience is a common one for bright, active girls with AD/HD. She functioned well enough to get along on the strength of her native ability, but spent many wasted years, underestimating her own intelligence and having no clear sense of direction. Looking back, Sally believes that more guidance and structure would have been of great benefit, but teachers and parents didn't expect much of her. It was only much later that she can to have higher expectations for herself.

Mary, portions of whose poem are included here, had a very different self-image than Susan. While Susan was physically active and competitive, the "tomboy" variety of AD/HD in girls, Mary was quiet, artistic and non-assertive. She had very little success in school and grew up believing herself to be "dumb." Now in her forties, Mary was recently diagnosed with AD/HD. She has only recently acknowledged her artistic ability. Mary is working hard to come to terms with who she is and to overcome the very low self-esteem from which she suffered during her school years.

School overwhelmed me
I couldn't understand

Just how to behave
To fit into their plan

The classes were long
I could not stay clear
My brain was so busy
Pretending to hear

I dreaded the clock
And its torturous pace
I could never keep up
I would just lose my place

For years I felt less than
With no self esteem
I thought I was stupid
Began to careen . . .

As Mary's poem continues, she describes her descent, during high school years, into promiscuity, desperately seeking a positive response from boys—the only arena where she experienced success.

Anne-Marie, like Mary, was also on the quiet, non-hyperactive side of the AD/HD equation, but presented a more complex and puzzling picture because she was able to excel, academically, in some areas. At the same time, however, Anne-Marie had enormous difficulty concentrating while reading. As a result, she rarely read books. She was so clearly capable and talented in music and writing that her reading difficulties were dismissed as "laziness."

"I was a quiet kid. No one really noticed me at school, apart from the ones that enjoyed reading my stories or my flute playing. I had trouble socializing with the other kids and stuck to one friend who was trustworthy. I was quiet, but sometimes, when I did open my mouth, I said the wrong thing.

School days were hell. I was bullied and didn't know how to stick up for myself. I could never find the right words. Although I was praised for my English essays, I struggled with comprehension. I loved stories, but I avoided books as I found it difficult to concentrate. My dad would often accuse me of being lazy because I didn't read.

All through school I felt ugly and stupid. However, I got through it because I thought I would grow out of it. I would constantly fantasize about the person I was going to be—Anne-Marie, the famous musician, Anne-Marie the record producer . . ."

Anne-Marie had big dreams, but mostly they were daydreams—with no concrete plan to implement them. She comforted herself with daydreams while she suffered from teasing, criticism and highly variable grades. And now, as a young adult, she remains stuck, drifting, full of self-recrimination.

Three different stories: Sally, the athletic tom boy, seen as having "average ability"; Mary, the quiet, shy girl who was "not very smart;" and Anne Marie, clearly talented in music and writing, but written off as "lazy" when her overall academic record did not match her recognized ability.

"Sweet, but not very bright; talented but 'lazy'; an 'average girl' who is doing 'just fine.' " Different explanations, but all three are classic ways that girls with AD/HD are diminished, and gradually learn to discount themselves and their abilities.

The parents' role

How can we prevent our daughters today from being dismissed in this fashion, and prevent them from underestimating themselves? Thom Hartmann, a widely read author on AD/HD, and father of two daughters with AD/HD, believes that one of the major reasons that girls are overlooked in schools has to do with the way that parents, with or without awareness, train their sons and daughters differently.

"In our culture we tell two stories, no matter how enlightened we may be. Little boys are told that if they have a need they should meet it in the environment. Boys are taught to acquire physical, interpersonal power, but little girls are told to internalize— "Sit down, be quiet, be a lady." Boys learn to reach out and grab when they need stimulation; girls learn how to achieve stimulation inside their own heads."

Whether we attribute the development of primarily inattentive type AD/HD behaviors to the socialization process that Thom Hartmann describes, or to inborn physiological, temperamental differences, our task as parents remains the same—to empower our daughters to ask for what they need, and to teach them that they are in school to learn and grow, not just to please the teacher and stay out of trouble!

How teachers can help with the identification process

Before girls with AD/HD can be helped, they must first be identified—not always an easy process. Just as a chameleon strives to hide, to blend in with its surroundings, to camouflage himself, so do many girls with AD/HD attempt a disappearing act in the classroom. It's no wonder that teachers often overlook them. They can be hard to spot—partly because many of them do not fit the standard AD/HD profile that teachers have been taught to recognize, and even harder because many girls go to great effort to escape their teacher's notice. An AD/HD-savvy teacher should be on the look-out for girls who:

- talk compulsively

- have difficulty following directions

- always seem to ask the student next to them what they're supposed to do

- sit quietly at their desk, but never seem to finish their assignments

- have desks, that are much messier than those of their classmates

- often forget to turn in permission slips, and leave homework at home

- frequently don't have all of the supplies they need in class

- look "attentive," but can't answer the question when called upon

- seem to have auditory processing problems

- seem to have expressive language problems

- have a slow response time

- tend to work very slowly

The legal/educational guidelines for AD/HD

The diagnosis of AD/HD is based upon diagnostic criteria established by the American Psychiatric Association. For a diagnosis of AD/HD to be made, these guidelines require that AD/HD can be shown to significantly impair her ability to function in a major life function, such as academic functioning, social functioning and functioning in daily life. In a psychological assessment, the impact of AD/HD upon academic functioning is typically measured by a discrepancy between her "potential," based on IQ, and her actual level of functioning. Thus, if a girl with a very high IQ functions in the average or even high average range in school, she still can be said to be significantly impacted by her AD/HD because her potential is so much higher than her performance.

In an educational setting, however, impairment is often measured against grade level performance rather than potential. A very bright girl, whose potential is at the 95th percentile, or higher, may not be seen as having an AD/HD-related impairment if she is able to function at grade level. Many women with AD/HD, diagnosed as adults, report that their high potential was unrecognized or overlooked, and their grade-level performance was seen as adequate. Worse yet, their grade-level performance was seen as all that they were capable of achieving!

It is also important that we don't place too much emphasis on academic functioning, ignoring the potential of AD/HD to have a very damaging effect upon the self-esteem and identity development of girls. The importance of this impact should not be overlooked, especially in girls whose enormous efforts to compensate for their AD/HD allows them to earn average or above average grades in school. Because the indicators are internalized, it's far too easy to miss the destructive impact to their self-esteem and to use their painfully earned grades as evidence that they have no need of academic support.

AD/HD among high academic performers

Despite the fact that evidence of academic difficulties is not the *sine qua non* of AD/HD, some professionals still mistakenly believe that one cannot succeed academically and yet have AD/HD. While hints of AD/HD may be present from early childhood, bright children, especially females who have been socialized to be more controlled and less disruptive within the classroom setting, may, in fact, be found among the top students in the early grades.

Often, in high school, AD/HD patterns become more evident as academic demands increase. But, a student may continue to make good grades, strictly on the basis of high intelligence, despite poor study habits, difficulty in concentrating while reading, inattention in class, and extreme procrastination when writing papers and completing projects.

It is, in fact, quite possible to earn doctoral, medical or law degrees, and yet have AD/HD, although many bright people fall along the wayside due to lack of diagnosis and treatment. Although supporting research is yet to be done, it seems likely that AD/HD is over-represented among doctoral degree candidates who have difficulty in completing their dissertations. What does this imply? Simply that one can be a good student throughout elementary and high school and yet have AD/HD. One can do well in college despite AD/HD, and can even go on to post-graduate education. And yet, regrettably, many parents are told that grade-level work renders their daughter ineligible for supports or accommodations along the way.

Achievement at the cost of extreme effort

In viewing the academic progression of girls with AD/HD, it is easy to forget the extreme effort often required of them to achieve these goals. The fact that they make these extreme efforts, often involving chronic anxiety, desperate all-night efforts, feelings of being overwhelmed, struggling as they try to write papers and complete projects, should not be used as evidence that they need no accommodations or assistance!

Parents who suspect that their daughter may have attentional problems should not rely solely upon the classroom teacher to make this identification. If the teacher or school does not recognize attentional difficulties in their daughter, they should seek a private evaluation from a professional who has experience in working with girls, and who recognizes the different histories and patterns that some girls demonstrate. Following a private diagnosis, they can then approach the school, asking for a teacher conference to discuss the findings and to request specific accommodations.

Parents need to educate themselves as much as possible about AD/HD, especially AD/HD in girls, and to keep in mind that they are pioneers in seeking accommodations for their daughters. They may have to play a strong advocacy and education role with the school. As teacher education regarding the different presentation of many girls with AD/HD expands, such strenuous parent advocacy may not remain necessary in the future.

When advocacy is not enough

Because girls with AD/HD often present differently, and with more internalizing disorders such as anxiety and depression, sometimes even ardent advocacy is not enough to gain the needed supports and accommodations.

—⁓⁓⁓—

"The modern classroom has proven basically toxic for Mindy. The exciting, noisy, visually stimulating, socially intense classroom we have today just overwhelms her. She is strong academically, yet performs inconsistently. Third grade has been catastrophic for her. A myriad of well-intentioned professionals can't fathom how someone can be very bright and very good in academic tasks and still have learning and attention differences severe enough to impair functioning. They also can't understand the toll taken even by successful coping mechanisms."

—⁓⁓⁓—

Mindy's mother makes a critical point here, for girls with AD/HD—the great, and typically hidden cost of coping mechanisms. Girls, out of an internal pressure to please, to do what is expected of them, make enormous efforts, for which they are sometimes, ironically "punished" through denial of accommodations. If a girl is able, with enormous effort, to meet grade level expectations, she is then found ineligible for accommodations and supports!

———∿∿∿———

"This year, even when she had the AD/HD diagnosis, had been taking Ritalin for 1.5 years, was getting informal accommodations, and was making daily visits to the clinic (just to get out of the stressful class) the local screening committee decided she was ineligible for a 504 plan because she was at or above grade level in all her academic subjects."

———∿∿∿———

Mindy's mother goes on to relate that her daughter's stress level led to increasing depression and anxiety. As stress escalated, Mindy reacted with panic, on occasion refusing to attend school. Ultimately, the school responded, not with a plan to accommodate her AD/HD, but with placement in a class for the emotionally disturbed. Mindy is unhappy in this class, and exhibits increasing depression. Ironically, her depression is interpreted as evidence that this class for the emotionally disturbed is the appropriate placement for her. Her parents and psychiatrist strongly disagree, because they see the "other" Mindy—*"the creative, compassionate, kind, strong, incredibly intelligent, incredibly lonely Mindy."* Both Mindy's mother and her psychiatrist strongly believe that her anxiety and depression are *secondary* to her AD/HD, and that what she needs are the structures and supports appropriate for a gifted child with AD/HD.

Mindy's troubling, story is an extreme example of difficulties that can be experienced by girls with AD/HD—who are more likely to be compliant, anxious, overwhelmed, and depressed. Inadequate supports for a sensitive, gifted girl with AD/HD have created a situation in which her secondary emotional reaction is seen as her primary diagnosis!

Helping classroom teachers to recognize and identify AD/HD in girls

As Thom Hartmann described, for many girls with AD/HD their disorder is an "internalized" one. While boys with AD/HD may "externalize" their needs—through demanding, arguing, fighting, resisting or disrupting, many girls do not manifest their needs and feelings externally. One of the best ways to find out about a girl's needs is to ask—in a setting where a girl can feel safe and secure. For girls age 10 and above, a self-report form may prove very beneficial, if the teacher notes any of the behavior patterns listed earlier in this chapter, suggestive of AD/HD. For girls under the age of 10, a verbal interview with the girl and her parent or parents may yield better information. A teacher should keep in mind that many girls won't "show" you, but, if she feels safe, she might "tell" you what is wrong.

Teachers can find a self-report questionnaire at the end of Chapter Four, as well as a list of questions at the end of each chapter from pre-school through high school. Teachers are encouraged to use these questionnaires as screening devices. While they are not diagnostic tools, they can be used very effectively as an initial screening. If a girl responds in the affirmative to a majority of the items, it may be appropriate to communicate to the parents that a full evaluation may be warranted.

What do they need from their teacher?

As with any student, their needs for support change when academic demands change as they move through elementary school to middle and high school. First, let's look at common needs across the age span of 6 through 18, and then, later, we'll highlight additional support needed in the upper grades.

Support and encouragement

One issue that girls with AD/HD describe, whether they fall on the hyperactive/hyper-social side or on the quiet, daydreamy side of AD/HD, is a sense of embarrassment or shame in the classroom. Some may deal with this feeling by showing an "attitude" of resentment ("The best defense is a good offense."); others by clowning and joking ("If I'm silly and entertaining, no one will notice that I never know what page we're on."); by ingratiating themselves to their teacher ("If she likes me, then maybe she won't get mad at me."); and still others by attempting to "disappear" ("If I hide, then I won't get in trouble."). Due to low self-esteem, self-blame and feelings of shame, what almost none of them do, is express their fears and embarrassment to their teacher. Without adequate explanation, the teacher is left to her own devices to understand why Sally is frequently absent from school, is never finished with her desk work, or is usually jabbering to the kid sitting next to her.

When a teacher acknowledges these types of behaviors, and recognizes that they may be suggestive of AD/HD, the most helpful response is one of encouragement and support. Rather than admonishing a girl for "not listening to directions," the AD/HD-sensitive teacher can give her explicit permission to quietly ask her neighbor what to do. The shy, withdrawn, insecure girl with AD/HD may be best placed next to a well-organized friend from whom she can ask assistance without embarrassment. A teacher can explicitly encourage these girls to come to him or her for extra support, and can more frequently cruise by her desk to redirect and encourage her.

An AD/HD-friendly classroom

❶ Make the classroom feel "safe"

In the most general sense, the teacher can give great support to AD/HD girls through making the classroom a comfort zone—where they can feel safe to make mistakes, to ask the teacher to repeat herself, or to explain that, yet again, she has forgotten to bring in her homework. Teachers who want to create a more AD/HD-friendly classroom can:

- Problem-solve with the student rather than criticize her for losing or forgetting something.

- Avoid calling on the shy, inattentive girl. Make a pact with her that she will be called upon only when she raises her hand, indicating that she knows the answer.

- Encourage her to come to the teacher's desk for a private explanation if she's feeling confused or unsure of how to proceed.

- Use encouragement and support, rather than admonishment and criticism to increase desired behaviors.

The more her teacher can recognize her curiosity, creativity and enthusiasm, and de-emphasize her forgetfulness, inattention or disorganization, the young female student with AD/HD can develop the building blocks of self-esteem which will help her develop into a confident young woman who believes in her own capabilities.

② Accommodate AD/HD to minimize its impact

- Seat the compulsive talker away from her best friends, letting her know that this is not meant as a punishment, but as a way to support her in getting her work done.

- Minimize the transporting of papers to and from school.

- Use the internet—to post homework assignments, list questions or problems for test review, and information for parents.

- Reduce the number of questions or assigned problems for students who have slow processing speed. Many students can adequately learn and can demonstrate that learning without completing as many items as have been assigned to the whole class.

- Allow re-taking of tests to accommodate the inconsistency of AD/HD performance. The goal of education is to learn and to be able to demonstrate that learning, not to pass or fail a test on a particular day.

- Don't mark off for messiness—while this may be a sign of decreased effort for students without AD/HD, poor handwriting, erasures and general messiness are hallmarks of AD/HD written work. The most constructive solution is the early development of keyboarding skills. It's much easier to push a key than to copy a letter of the alphabet, and "erasures" on the computer screen are invisible, allowing the student with AD/HD to eventually produce a neat, legible product.

- Give students with AD/HD stronger encouragement to develop keyboarding skills by making daily keyboarding practice a routine for them in the classroom. Fifteen minutes a day with a keyboarding program can help a child to rapidly progress in keyboarding skills.

- Recognize that daydreaming is often beyond her control. Draw her back to attention discretely, without teasing or criticizing.

- Lecture for shorter periods of time and engage all of your students, AD/HD or not, through more class discussion and interaction.

- Recognize that transitions can be difficult for her. She may have become so involved in one activity that she doesn't hear you tell the class that it's time for another subject.

- Recognize that a child with AD/HD can appear inconsiderate despite her very real concern for others.

Accommodations for girls in the upper grades

As girls move from elementary to middle and high school, challenges increase and life becomes increasingly complex.

The need for accommodations and services is typically much greater during these years because:

1. Girls move from a single teacher to multiple teachers

2. Homework assignments and reading requirements lengthen

3. Demands for organization greatly increase

4. Social pressures increase and become more complex as boy/girl relationships come into the picture, social cliques form, and one's identity is increasingly dependent upon social groups and extracurricular activities

5. Progression into adolescence increases expectations that girls should generally be able to function more independent of structure and guidance provided by parents and teachers

6. Hormonal changes and fluctuations tend to increase mood lability and to intensify the impact of AD/HD patterns

Classroom/teacher accommodations appropriate in upper grades

- A note-taker (or access to the teacher's notes) for class lectures so that the student can listen and interact without needing to simultaneously take detailed notes.

- Extended time on tests.

- Provision of a separate, quiet room in which to take tests.

- Alternative forms of tests, including essay tests and oral examinations

- Reasonable flexibility in meeting deadlines

- Extra text books available in the classroom for times when the text may have been accidentally left at home or in the locker

- Internet posting of homework assignments, guidelines for long-term assignments, and dates of upcoming quizzes, tests and due dates of papers and projects.

(It is important for high school teachers to be aware that *all* of these accommodations, aside from extra textbooks, are typically available on the college campus, and are needed even more on the high school level.)

School-wide supports for girls with AD/HD

What kind of supports should the school offer as girls move from the classroom cocoon of elementary school to the relative independence of middle and high school?

① Recognition that their need for support is ongoing, and is likely to continue into adulthood

Many teachers feel that it is their mandate, when working with adolescent students, to prepare them for independent living after high school. They repeatedly give students messages about the "real world" after high school, admonishing them that there will be no one to remind them, to organize them or to guide them, and that they need to practice and prepare for this imminent state of independence. What these teachers often don't realize is that students with AD/HD will continue to struggle with problems of forgetfulness, distractibility and disorganization throughout their lives. The goal of independent living, without supports, in adulthood is neither necessary nor realistic for all adults with AD/HD. In fact, feeling the pressure to achieve these goals often triggers feelings of demoralization or hopelessness. An important aspect of success as an adult with AD/HD is learning how to find and surround oneself with the supports necessary to function well. High school is the place to begin to identify and put these types of support into place. Many of these students will need organizational supports in high school, in college, and in the workplace as adults, as well as in their personal lives.

The challenge for middle and high school teachers is to provide structure and support for students with AD/HD while encouraging them to develop independence in areas in which they are capable.

② Provision of an AD/HD counselor/coach

As students with AD/HD move from a single teacher in elementary school, to multiple teachers in middle and high school, they will greatly benefit from having one person with whom they can check in on a frequent basis. This advisor/coach/counselor can help them learn to schedule, prioritize and organize the multiple demands from multiple teachers. While the need for such coaching and study skills training has been recognized and often provided on the college level, most middle and high schools do not yet offer the services of such a support person.

❸ School-based support groups

Girls with AD/HD, much more frequently than boys with AD/HD, report feeling socially isolated, "different" from their peers, and very unhappy in this isolation. Most AD/HD interventions focus on academic support, and on methods to control rebellious or antagonistic behavior, with little attention paid to the social anxieties that are of such great concern for girls with AD/HD.

The best way that we can help inoculate these girls against feeling like social misfits is to help them to develop interests and talents, to help them feel a sense of commonality with other girls struggling with similar issues, and to give them positive role models. A girls' support group, headed by a school counselor or psychologist is an ideal way to provide such support.

❹ Priority, customized registration

Rising at an early hour to concentrate in seven different classes during a long, tiring and distracting day is a challenge for all adolescents, but often poses an all but impossible challenge for teens with AD/HD. One of the most important ways that schools can accommodate the teen with AD/HD is to customize her registration so that her most challenging classes are taught at optimal times of day, with less challenging classes interspersed among those which are most challenging for her. If she is provided with an AD/HD counselor or coach in the middle and high school level, someone who knows her strengths and weaknesses, this is the ideal person to help her arrange for customized registration at the beginning of each term. Colleges and universities very commonly provide priority registration to students with AD/HD, however very few middle and high schools have instituted similar policies.

⑤ Self-advocacy training

All students with AD/HD need to make the successful transition from a dependency upon parental advocacy to advocating for their own educational needs. Girls with AD/HD have a special need to learn self-advocacy because of their strong tendency to hide, to be self-effacing, to feel too embarrassed or threatened to make their needs known. Girls who have hidden for years in elementary school, depending upon their mother to talk to their teachers and counselors, have a long journey to reach the point that they can successfully advocate for themselves, especially as they encounter skeptical or non-supportive teachers in high school and beyond.

Unfortunately, many high school counselors emphasize the need for self-advocacy without providing any training to make it possible. And girls, who have been taught since earliest childhood, to accommodate, to adapt, to internalize—have a much greater challenge than their male counterparts in learning to speak up for themselves. A girls' AD/HD support group could also provide an excellent setting in which to develop these advocacy skills.

Alternatives to public school

Private schools

One alternative to public schools, albeit an expensive one, is to find a private school setting which is more appropriate to the needs of the girl with AD/HD. Because girls with AD/HD are diverse, the ideal academic setting for one girl may actually be inappropriate for another. Parents, whose budgets allow, may benefit from seeking the assistance of a school placement specialist in selecting a school. Some girls with AD/HD, especially those of the shy, inattentive type, may thrive in a school that offers small class size and a very personalized, supportive teaching style. Others may thrive in a highly structured school setting that offers supervised study periods and structured help in learning to plan and to organize. Yet some girls may find such a setting too controlling and confining, and may thrive in a school that emphasizes creativity and independence. A few very bright girls with AD/HD may not qualify for gifted programs within the public school system due to mediocre grades. However, a private school that recognizes their talents and can challenge them academically may allow a girl with high IQ to feel more stimulated and motivated. Some private schools are in a better position to individualize the teaching approach and academic requirements to suit the needs of the student.

Lisa was identified with AD/HD in elementary school. She was strong-willed, emotionally reactive and hyper-talkative. When AD/HD was mentioned, teachers and principals responded that she performed above grade-level, but was a discipline problem at times. Her parents were admonished to provide more structure and discipline at home. A private evaluation revealed an IQ at the 99th percentile, an ability level that certainly wasn't reflected in Lisa's school performance.

As Lisa entered middle school, then high school, her performance declined. She felt lost in large classes. Her hyper-social, hyper-talkative nature led teachers to react with annoyance. When her parents requested school conferences to discuss her special needs, they were admonished for Lisa's irresponsibility and lack of discipline.

Despite increasing academic difficulties, Lisa intensely resisted the idea of a private school. At ages 13, 14 and 15 her social world defined her. Finally, in her sophomore year of high school, Lisa herself began to realize that she was throwing away her future by remaining in a school that couldn't meet her needs. Despite the painful social upheaval, Lisa agreed that she needed to remove herself from public school and from the temptations of her social life. She entered a private boarding school that offered a class size of 8 or 10, that provided a structured study hall each evening, and that gave her a daily tutoring session to help her with planning, organization and assistance with writing assignments.

Now a student at a competitive university, she receives excellent academic supports for AD/HD and LD. As Lisa looks back, she believes that she would never have gone on to success in college without the supports she received in boarding school. Rather than languishing in public high school as a very bright girl who earned mediocre grades, she received the support that allowed her to work up to her potential.

———— ∽∽∽ ————

Home schooling

Home schooling is becoming an alternative that is opted for increasingly as families are frustrated by the low morale and academic struggles that their daughters with AD/HD experience in a public school setting.

Home schooling is not for every family, however, and needs

to be carefully considered. For home schooling to be successful, the girl with AD/HD needs to live in a home that provides the necessary structure and support for her to succeed, or needs to be highly self-motivated. Even when home schooling is successful on an academic level, parents need to be careful to balance their daughter's activities so that she does not become socially isolated, and so that she has the opportunity to participate in the extra-curricular activities available to students in the public schools.

Many parents have found a balance between the advantages of home schooling and the opportunities available in public schools by arranging with the local public school for their child to participate in physical education, music, art, and after school clubs and sports. There are a number of structured programs that have been developed to help parents follow a home schooling program for their child that will prepare her across the broad range of academic subjects that are typically covered by the public schools.

This home schooling story comes from a family of three children with AD/HD. Their second child, a daughter, was on the quiet, less assertive side. She did well in elementary school, where she had the benefit of small classes, but began to fall apart as she entered her junior and senior years of high school. As their second daughter, and youngest child followed along, her AD/HD was easier to identify. Kay was more assertive and outgoing, like her older brother. Her parents felt that they had overlooked so much with her sister, and were careful not to make the same mistake twice.

Several weeks after Kay entered the new, large public high school, she was coming home angry on a daily basis—complaining of senseless rules, of boring classes and indifferent teachers. As her misery increased week by week, her parents took note. After an especially explosive confrontation between the students and faculty about behavior in the halls between classes, Kay came home announcing that she wanted to try home schooling. Although her parents voiced some doubts, they did not want her to repeat the pattern of frustration and failure of her older sister.

The family launched into unfamiliar territory with their youngest child. Kay, who had always been encouraged to think and act independently, researched an internet based home school program, and, with her parents' permission, enrolled. Four years later, Kay relates:

"My friends laughed at me when I told them I decided I was going to homeschool. I was tired of weekly meetings with my teachers (to discuss problems), of sitting in class seven hours a day, of not being with my friends. In homeschooling I could go at my own pace. My teachers were patient with me and gave me the time to finish my work. They gave me the responsibility to finish it, and had complete trust that I would get it done. Another thing is that many of my activities were hands-on. For one social studies project my mother and I visited a non-profit agency where I learned how dogs are trained to lead blind people.

As I explored more in depth with homeschooling I began to realize that learning was, for myself, bringing out those qualities and talents within myself. I discovered how certain herbs help different parts of the human body. I wrote poetry and short stories. I looked for whatever made my blood sizzle and I did that.

*Right now I'm at a two-year college studying
various courses to get my two-year degree. Homeschooling led me to where I am right now and it was
the best decision I've ever made."*

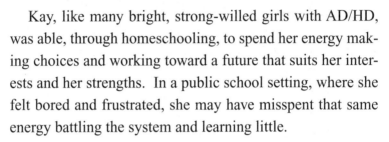

Kay, like many bright, strong-willed girls with AD/HD,
was able, through homeschooling, to spend her energy making choices and working toward a future that suits her interests and her strengths. In a public school setting, where she
felt bored and frustrated, she may have misspent that same
energy battling the system and learning little.

Homeschooling certainly isn't for every family, or for every student with AD/HD, but it offers the possibility of providing both the structure and the flexibility which are so often the key for success as a student with AD/HD.

Bringing in other professionals to support girls with AD/HD

Ideally, all of the necessary academic supports would be provided for girls with AD/HD by the public school system. But,
realistically, this is unlikely to happen.

Parents of girls with AD/HD need to work hard to bring
the public school system into the loop in recognizing and
helping their daughter with AD/HD, but should not expect
that all needs can or will be met at school.

Educational diagnostician

As has been mentioned earlier, when parents suspect that
their daughter may have AD/HD, but the teacher(s) do not

recognize a problem, perhaps their best option is to elect to have their daughter evaluated by a private expert in the area of AD/HD. This individual may be a clinical psychologist, a neuro-psychologist or an educational diagnostician. While the testing should contain standard, well-recognized tests in order to document an AD/HD diagnosis, the most critical and useful part of the test report is the list of recommendations regarding treatment, educational needs and accommodations. The parent can then return to the school with a documented disability and commence the process by which an individual educational plan (I.E.P.) or "504" plan (so called because of Section 504 of the Rehabilitation Act) can be developed to meet their daughter's educational needs in the school system. Often it can be helpful if the professional who conducted the evaluation accompanies the parent to the school meeting, to explain and discuss the recommendations in the report.

Tutor

AD/HD traits, combined with years of self-doubts and low self-esteem, can lead girls with AD/HD to shy away from challenging courses, or to assume, if such courses are required, that they will do poorly in them. Even when there is no evidence of a learning disability in a particular subject, a girl with AD/HD may greatly benefit from working one-on-one with a tutor. A tutor can support girls with AD/HD in particular areas of weakness such as math, written language, or memory. She can also help her to develop the organizational and general study skills she'll need as academic demands increase in middle and high school.

Coach

Even when a girl with AD/HD is bright enough to compensate academically, her AD/HD may impact her in profound ways that make school highly stressful.

———⁓⁓⁓———

"My daughter, 13, is mind-bogglingly brilliant; she knocks the top off of every standardized test, with seventh grade college board scores of over 1200, but is unable to keep track of assignments, notebooks, lab work. She is so disorganized that we have to make a special trip to empty out her locker once a week, so she'll have a coat or sweatshirt for the following Monday."

———⁓⁓⁓———

A girl like this could greatly benefit from specialized coaching that can help her to become better organized and less forgetful. Coaching, unlike tutoring, focuses on setting concrete goals such as habit development, and supporting the girl to follow-through on a daily basis until habits of planning and organization have become established.

Coaching for children and teens with AD/HD is a newly emerging profession that shows great promise as a tool to help students compensate for typical AD/HD patterns of disorganization and forgetfulness.

Conclusion

The responsibility falls upon parents of daughters with AD/HD to try to ensure that they receive the educational support that they need and that their full potential is reached. Parents must first become strong advocates for their daughters and teach their daughters to become strong advocates for themselves. As we've seen in the several clinical vignettes introduced in this chapter, sometimes even strong advocacy within the public school system will not suffice. Some families will choose to opt for alternatives, either private schooling or home schooling, to avoid potentially damaging situations.

The most critical issue for girls with AD/HD is to become identified so that they may receive the appropriate support, accommodations and treatment. The potential of so many girls is wasted because they are dismissed or overlooked. Teachers, very understandably, will have a more difficult time identifying the less-obvious behaviors of many girls with AD/HD. Girls with AD/HD who are functioning on grade level, but whose potential is far above their peers, are likely to be overlooked in a public school system which already feels stretched beyond capacity in its attempt to meet the diverse needs of many students. Much more professional, teacher and parent education is necessary before the identification and adequate accommodation and support of girls with AD/HD becomes routine in our public classrooms.

Chapter Ten

Treatment Approaches

I t is clear by now that AD/HD is a complex condition that pervades every aspect of a girl's life. It makes sense, then, that the management of AD/HD must be approached on every possible front to address the overt symptoms as well as the subtler manifestations. Marcel Kinsbourne, M.D., summarized it best when he wrote, "AD/HD management should constitute a prime example of treatment targeted on quality-of-life considerations." (Kinsbourne, 1992). He points to the overemphasis on the management of AD/HD for improved school behavior and performance as short-sighted. Quality-of-life issues that have an even greater impact on a child's life are daily interactions with parents, siblings, and extended family. Repeated negative interactions, that are gradually internalized into a girl's identity and can permanently damage self-esteem, are critical concerns. It is essential that a girl with AD/HD feel able to express her thoughts and feelings accurately, and to respond appropriately and assertively in order to have her needs met.

Catch it early

Early intervention is the key to successful AD/HD treatment. Since AD/HD is a neurophysiological difference that likely has been present since birth, as soon as AD/HD is suspected, it should be investigated. Early intervention is the insurance that non-adaptive coping patterns will not become entrenched, and that co-existing symptoms will be less likely to develop secondary to the AD/HD. Above all, the earlier that identification and intervention can begin, the less damage will be done to a girl's developing sense of self.

Learning about AD/HD

Gaining a working knowledge of AD/HD is the single most essential factor in its successful management. An in-depth understanding of the diagnosis and its impact provides a context for interpreting non-adaptive behaviors that sometimes seem to defy logic. The girl, as well as her parents, siblings, extended family and teachers, all need to appreciate the multi-faceted fallout that may result due to this chronic struggle. As they gather insight into the often-frustrating behaviors otherwise deemed "intentional," accusations and anger will gradually yield to feelings of tolerance, support and compassion.

As negative feedback decreases, sadness and shame will decrease, and the girl's damaged sense of self can begin to heal. The optimum AD/HD-friendly education includes the proviso that understanding offers an explanation, but not an excuse. Girls need to be taught that it's not their "fault," but it *is* their responsibility to learn strategies to meet the challenges of AD/HD.

Parent advocacy

This journey of "psychoeducation" is generally pursued by the girl's parents, often guided by a professional, and can include any of the wide range of resources available on the topic, including articles, books, videos, websites, workshops, conferences, and support organizations. As the parents learn about the unique ways in which AD/HD manifests itself in their daughter, they are in the best position to communicate this knowledge to her teachers. Parents need to understand that this task falls upon their shoulders; they are the only ones who can alert the teachers, guidance counselors and administrators to her special needs. Until she can advocate for herself, no one will advocate for your daughter unless you do. And before you begin—know the laws (see Chapter Nine).

Many parents speak with the teachers of the core academic subjects; however, it is also prudent to speak with the teachers of special subjects (art, music, gym, computers, and so on). Some feel that this is unnecessary, but because these are the more novel and less structured activities, their less predictable format can be especially challenging for a girl with AD/HD. In fact, these are just the environments in which interactions take place most freely, and can careen off-course most easily. It is helpful to maintain the perspective that damaged self-esteem is a far greater tragedy than a damaged GPA.

In addition to initially informing the teachers and administration, open communication and regular consultations will keep parents abreast of behavioral and academic performance trends. In that way, problems can be identified and discussed, within an AD/HD framework, before they escalate. Never assume that you will get a call if there is a "problem"; your definition of a problem and a teacher's definition of a problem may differ, since you each have different expectations and goals for your daughter.

Developmentally, it is a slow and gradual process for children to gain complete facility with verbal communication. Especially when they are under stress, children naturally regress, and resort to behavior to communicate. With this in mind, when you, as parent or teacher, are confronted by a difficult-to-manage behavior, it can be helpful to ask yourself, "What is she trying to tell me?"

We do not to want to, in any way, minimize the extraordinary frustration that arises in the face of these behaviors. Yet, the more that adults can be empathetic, and see a struggling child when they hear a defiant comment, the more hope there is for the girl's self-esteem to remain intact. That understanding, which will help to diffuse anger, requires serious work, and is usually achieved by a parent first. It is then the parent's job to reframe their daughter's behavior in this way for the teachers. It is essential for everyone involved to remember that a negative statement, whether made by a peer, teacher, or parent, has the same devastating impact on a fragile ego.

Individual therapy

While the core symptoms of AD/HD are neurobiologically based, and cannot be altered significantly by general psychotherapy, specialized types of therapy can be very helpful in addressing the constellation of issues that encircle this core.

Integrating numerous schools of thought, therapy approaches focus on real-life issues and work toward setting goals using concrete strategies, and monitoring progress. In addition, the feelings that accompany the struggle are discussed, so that the interplay of psychological and neurological understanding can be used to advantage. Also, numerous coexisting conditions respond well to psychotherapy, as do emotional issues such as low self-esteem and shame.

In addition to addressing problem-solving issues and coexisting disorders, many girls find it useful and comforting to be able to share their feelings and concerns as they process their understanding of AD/HD. Individual treatment can be extremely useful as a means of helping the girl reframe her symptoms in a more positive light.

While it is critical to acknowledge the ways in which AD/HD makes daily functioning a challenge, it is equally important to embrace the strengths that will get these girls to their goals. The critical issue is to choose a therapist who truly understands the nuances of AD/HD in girls, and utilizes a strengths-based assessment; often, a woman therapist is the best choice for a girl. Of these therapists, most will work simultaneously on practical problem solving around issues with family, peers, school, organizations, etc.—and on the underlying emotional issues as well.

Heidi tearfully separated from her father, following a fun-filled weekend visit. Her mother tried to comfort her with hugs and kisses. While sensation-craving girls with AD/HD would likely welcome such an expression of affection, this was experienced as a

*sensation overload for Heidi. She found the close-
ness intrusive, and it made her feel even worse.*

*In therapy, Heidi brought up this issue, saying that
she was feeling guilty about how angry she got at her
mother when she came home, especially after not seeing her for the whole weekend. As the scenario was
explored, the therapist helped Heidi to identify that
she and her mother expressed missing each other in
different ways. Heidi was already feeling fragile from
having to leave her father, and the neurological irritability triggered by her mother's physical closeness
made her cringe.*

*Heidi was happy to understand that she didn't
resent her mother, or love her father more. She began
to appreciate that transitions were difficult for her,
and that noticing how transitions were handled was
important information for her. In addition, she felt
empowered because she and her therapist developed
ways to let her mother know that, while she certainly
loved her, she preferred not to be hugged; she was
able to confidently explain that what she actually
needed was some quiet downtime when she came
home.*

*Heidi's mom, who had been feeling terribly re-
jected, welcomed the insights into her daughter's experience, and was happy to have an intervention that
she knew would ease the transition. The next time
that Heidi returned from a weekend with her father,
her mother showed her that she had set up a snack
for her next to the Nintendo. Then her mother kissed
her hair lightly as she left the room, and Heidi ea-
gerly sat down to play, easing into the warmth of being home with Mom.*

Group treatment

For girls with AD/HD, one of the most important therapeutic interventions is group treatment. Many AD/HD symptoms emerge when there are demands to process a lot of stimulation at the same time. In the controlled low-stimulation environment of individual treatment, situations that trigger distractibility or over-excitability rarely arise, making it difficult to practice new coping skills for these problems. It is the stressful classroom, recess, or the bus ride home that are times of potential disaster.

A group treatment situation can serve as a safe microcosm of the social situations that a girl with AD/HD faces. A great advantage is that a girl with AD/HD, who may be unaware of her impact on others, can actually witness how AD/HD behaviors affect others, by observing interactions among the group members. She can think through these issues much more clearly if she is not directly involved in the interaction.

In her own interactions with group members, any of the peer members or the group leader can point out problematic behavior patterns. This concept is particularly well suited to girls who understand themselves best in terms of their relation to others. For some girls with AD/HD, group therapy may represent one of the first social groups to which they have belonged and in which they have been truly accepted. Being a group member can help to normalize the experience of having AD/HD by demonstrating that her peers struggle with the same issues. The group also can validate a girl's experience as no individual therapist can, and that becomes a message that builds confidence. After Julia's second group session, she told her mother, "So it's not that I'm so weird. It's just that you do things differently with AD/HD, and now

I see how everybody with AD/HD deals with it."

The group also provides a safe forum for practicing skills related to social interaction, anger management, initiating conversation, and so on. Concrete strategies geared toward behavioral change are taught, such as planned situations, contingency management, modeling, cognitive behavioral techniques to improve self-monitoring, and positive self-talk (Holloway, L, 1999). Parents are also taught these techniques so that the family system can work together toward the same goals.

Since group work is situationally based, the therapist can intervene at the moment of difficulty and offer concrete coping suggestions that are relevant for all group members. The group can also brainstorm alternate solutions to a problem, and the members can learn from one another. Most girls with AD/HD find that it is rewarding to have their suggestions seriously respected and considered. Every girl will feel empowered by the experience of teaching her peers something valuable. The girl having difficulty can try out these solutions and gain immediate positive reinforcement for her attempts. Gradually, she will be able to accept responsibility for her behaviors, and can begin to generalize them to situations outside the therapy room.

Behavior modification

The main principle of behavioral treatment is that a girl's behavior can be altered by consistent, expected consequences administered directly following her behavior. Positive consequences, like praise and attention, will quickly reinforce behaviors that parents want to encourage. Negative consequences, like time-outs or loss of a privilege, will reduce the likelihood of repeated unwanted behavior. The parents, with the therapist's advice, will agree on and establish a set of clear and effective rules for behavioral expectation.

They will create an explicit list of behavioral expectations, consequences for failing to conform, and a reward system for successes. All of these conditions must be explained to the girl by both partners, and she must be given an opportunity for input. Some families prefer to write out the specifics as a contract, which all parties must sign; this step convinces some children to take the process more seriously.

The theory behind this system is that, when parents are well-armed with definitive consequences for specific behaviors, they can feel prepared to cope with the problem. Feeling confident about how to proceed confirms that the parent is indeed in control. Knowing you are in control removes the element of a power struggle with your daughter, and allows the parent to communicate in a more matter-of-fact way. Diffusing the intense anger that is evoked in a power struggle is a central goal of this system. By lowering the frustration level, the system can assist the parent in avoiding harsh and unrealistic punishments like "No TV for a month!" This system actually provides predictable structure for limit-setting and discipline, which works to everyone's advantage.

These techniques are logical, straightforward and seemingly simple when first described. However, putting these techniques into practice takes time, planning, patience, self-reflection, and a lot of hard work on the parents' part. Parents are always initially dubious when the psychologist tells them that this system will work. The only condition is that both parents must be completely consistent in administering the system—at home, in public, when you're tired or ill, when your child is pleading with you or crying hysterically. This is the part of the system that is extremely challenging, and requires both partners to be equally invested in making it work. It is also important to ensure that siblings, nannies, teachers and grandparents are all familiar with the system, so that the girl will receive a consistent message, wherever she is.

While positive results emerge relatively quickly, it is important to remember that children with AD/HD tend to need to practice the system more than other children might. Clearly, if one or both parents have AD/HD themselves, organizing and maintaining the system can be most difficult. If a parent with AD/HD is feeling overwhelmed with anger, try to count to ten before speaking. This will provide time to remember the system, access the appropriate consequences, and avoid saying something you might regret. Also, regardless of how enjoyable a task you are involved in when the rules are violated, you must act immediately; however inconvenient it may be; the shortest possible gap between the behavior and the statement of the consequence is a factor that can maximize success.

For example, when a girl successfully puts away all of her crayons and markers after using them, the parent or teacher can say, "What a responsible job you did putting away the art supplies!" This explicit and situation-specific praise (as opposed to "Good girl!"), accompanied by a smile and a discreet touch on the shoulder, is actually a very powerful reinforcement strategy. It provides a positive cue along three of the senses: the verbal statement she hears, the visual impact of the smile, the tactile touch on the shoulder. This multi-sensory statement is less likely to be missed, because so many senses are involved in processing the one communication.

For negative behaviors that aren't explicitly listed in your system, a parent can discipline her by putting her in a time-out. This involves establishing a quiet, safe, non-stimulating place in the house (stairways often work) where she can be sent to cool down for an agreed-upon length of time while being deprived of family interaction and stimulation. Generally, being deprived of the parent's attention is one of the best motivators for children with AD/HD.

Classroom interventions, school accommodations and tutoring

There are many modifications that can maximize a girl's academic performance while minimizing behavioral interference. However, it has recently been shown that a girls are more than three times as likely as boys to have unmet service needs (Bussing et al., 1998). An awareness of the educational options and rights for children with AD/HD can make advocacy attempts more effective. A full discussion of these educational interventions can be found in Chapter Nine.

Medication

It is widely accepted now that medication can dramatically improve many of the symptoms of AD/HD in many children. AD/HD symptoms are the result of imbalances or insufficiencies in the neurotransmitter chemicals in the brain, particularly the dopamine system. Medication can address these neurochemical imbalances so that the girl can function better. Medication cannot cure AD/HD, but it can improve the symptoms while it is working. Medication does not control the child, but rather allows the child to have more control over how she functions and who she can be. See Chapter 11 for a full discussion of pharmacological treatment for AD/HD girls.

Coaching

A coach can work one-on-one with a girl on a regular basis to help her reach her goals. Coaching is a partnership with someone who can help her learn to do the things she needs to do. A coach can help her become aware of how she functions, learns, manages her time, and make choices. Then, utilizing this unique profile of her strengths and weaknesses, the coach can help her expand her repertoire of automatic behaviors by providing the opportunity for consistent supervised practice of skills. A coach, whether in person or over the phone, gets involved on the nitty-gritty level and helps her with the executive functioning difficulties that are so central to AD/HD: planning her time, setting priorities, organizing assignments, breaking down tasks, and developing effective study skills. In addition, a coach serves as a cheerleader, sounding board, as well as provider of detailed constructive feedback.

For teens, a coach also can help to develop a set of long-range goals, as well as explicit plans for meeting those goals. After identifying a girl's personal roadblocks to success, a coach also will work on self-advocacy skills. When the struggle between parent and daughter over academics or other responsibilities becomes a central and harrowing aspect of their relationship, it is time to consider ways for the parent to divest herself of some of the centrality of her role. A coach can perform many of the skills-training and supervisory functions of a parent, without the intense emotional investment. In that way, a coach can broaden the support network and enlarge the safety net so that the parent-child relationship can become less control-oriented and more rewarding.

"Wrap-around" programs

A multi-modal treatment plan can be enhanced by "wrapping" intensive outpatient services around the child and her family. This enables a community agency to create continuity of care from school to home. This type of intervention is indicated when there are serious co-existing conditions that make management without external support difficult for a parent.

Alternative treatments

There are probably few parents who do not, initially, have concerns about giving medication to their young daughters. Most parents are reluctant to make that leap, and search for answers that may be more natural in origin. It is important for parents to be aware that there are few, if any, well-controlled studies of many of these alternative approaches, and the majority of AD/HD professionals maintain that there is no evidence that any of these techniques consistently improve AD/HD symptoms. However, there is such a wealth of anecdotal evidence regarding successful results that most parents are tempted and confused by the options.

The mechanisms by which medications work is not entirely clear, and they don't work for everybody. Each girl's brain and body will respond uniquely to the various possible interventions, and no one can predict where success will be found. At this point, perhaps you are considering whether or not one of these alternative treatments will help your daughter. It is important to remember that natural substances also have the risk of adverse side effects, just like medications. Also, most of these approaches also require an investment in the form of time, energy, and money. Parents should not abandon a treatment program that works for their daughter in order to pursue one of the alternatives. Here is an alphabetical list of some of the alternative approaches, along with a brief description of each:

Applied Kinesiology—chiropractic method of manipulating the cranial bones to achieve an alignment that allows sensory messages to flow uninterrupted.

Biofeedback—EEG training to increase brain waves associated with sustained attention, and decrease those associated with distractibility.

Treatment for Candida—medication and diet designed to discourage yeast overgrowth in the body, which may weaken the immune system, making it more susceptible to AD/HD symptoms.

Feingold Diet—a strict sugar and additive-free diet designed to eliminate food allergens that may induce symptoms mimicking AD/HD.

Inner Ear Dysfunction Treatment—a treatment attempting to re-establish vestibular balance with various medications (for example, motion-sickness drugs) to improve sensory integration and body energy.

Irlen Lenses—tinted lenses that filter certain wavelengths of light that may improve Scotopic Sensitivity Syndrome, which may mimic AD/HD symptoms.

Neuro-Linguistic Programming—a communication model used by professionals to enhance their ability to assist others in making positive changes by creating empowering and therapeutic environments.

Optometric Vision Training—exercises designed by optometrists to improve visual skills that may impact reading/learning problems.

Pycnogenol—a grape seed extract available in natural food stores that may improve focus.

Sensory-Motor Integration—exercises designed to help a child overcome individual sensitivities.

Super Blue-Green Algae—algae available through sales companies that may improve AD/HD symptoms by increasing the amount of oxygen available to the brain.

Treatment plans must consider co-existing disorders

Generally, the later a girl is diagnosed, the more likely it is that she will suffer from some type of emotional or psychiatric difficulty, in addition to the AD/HD. Psychiatric or developmental conditions coexisting with AD/HD are quite common, existing in almost 50% of children with AD/HD (Biederman et al., 1999). These "co-existing" disorders can alter the symptoms, pattern, course, treatment, and prognosis for a girl's AD/HD. Since other disorders can confound the presentation of symptoms, one disorder may be more obvious than another, and the full diagnosis may emerge over a period of time in treatment.

The tendency to internalize symptoms makes AD/HD girls more prone to develop a co-existing disorder, which can include mood disorders like depression, anxiety disorders and somatization disorders. For many girls, a history of chronic social and academic failure often leads to an escalating pattern of low self-esteem, irritability, demoralization, and learned helplessness.

Mood disorders

Co-existing mood disorders in girls are common, especially

if there is a family history of depression. The likelihood of developing such a disorder increases dramatically in the adolescent years, especially in the case of the primarily inattentive subtype, which can so easily evade detection. If the AD/HD remains untreated until the teen years, girls seeking help for their unhappiness may present with the symptoms of anxiety or depression, which may be easier to spot than the AD/HD symptoms. It is still common to find girls with undiagnosed AD/HD treated for an extended time for these coexisting diagnoses, without success. At this point in time, it is still a rare clinician that will then consider an AD/HD diagnosis.

Anxiety disorders

Anxiety disorders are another common co-existing condition for girls with AD/HD, especially in the Predominantly Inattentive subtype. Anxiety may express itself as separation anxiety, panic attacks, overanxious or avoidant disorder; social phobia or other specific phobias, or obsessive compulsive disorder. Furthermore, expressions of anxiety can change form throughout the developmental process; for example, separation anxiety in early childhood can be experienced as panic attacks as a teen, who may become a socially phobic adult. Anxiety and mood disorders can coexist along with the AD/HD diagnosis. In some cases, the stimulant medication often used to treat AD/HD symptoms can exacerbate anxiety symptoms; in other cases, the stimulant may produce symptoms of agitation and jitteriness that may be confused with an anxiety disorder. Somatization disorders are quite common in AD/HD girls, and are often expressed as gastrointestinal complaints and/or headaches.

Disruptive behavior disorders

While the Disruptive Behavior Disorders, besides AD/HD, are another major source of complications, they are more common in boys. Oppositional defiant disorder (ODD) is found in girls with AD/HD, though to a lesser extent than in boys, and is associated with an increased risk of behavioral, academic, and interpersonal difficulties. The AD/HD/ODD combination is among the more difficult cases to address—at home, in school and in treatment; interestingly, this also is a disorder that is characterized by "un-lady-like" behavior, which may render it even more distressing to parents and teachers. For example, if you ask your daughter to clean her room, a girl with AD/HD might "not hear you" or might "forget" or might say "I'll do it later." If you ask a girl with AD/HD and ODD to clean her room, she might say, "Do it yourself if you don't like it," or "Get out of here, it's private, and none of your business." They often refuse to take responsibility for their actions, and instead externalize the blame onto someone else: "I didn't break that glass. Timmy did it, he always breaks everything. He's a liar and you always blame me!" Anger exudes from these girls, and the intensity of this feeling, like all feelings, is amplified by the AD/HD.

While these types of interactions are painful and challenging, there are several steps that frustrated parents can take to reduce the level of tension in their homes. First, therapists can help families create highly structured behavioral systems discussed previously.

Another helpful move is to include an AD/HD coach in the family's support network. Often, oppositional girls with AD/HD respond most intensely to their parents, and can be far more reasonable with other authority figures, especially if there is a good fit in terms of personality styles. If the coach is responsible for working with the girl on homework and organizational issues, it diffuses the struggle between parent and child. In this way, parent and daughter are freed to have some fun interactions, where parents don't feel that they are in the role of "policeman," and where the daughter doesn't feel that she needs to be on the defensive. Another option is a trial of medicaton, which is discussed in Chapter 11.

Conduct disorder

Conduct disorder is seen even more rarely in girls with AD/HD, and involves serious antisocial behaviors such as aggression, lying, stealing, and truancy. While the oppositional defiant diagnosis always precedes the development of conduct disorder, an oppositional defiant disorder in the great majority of cases does not lead to conduct disorder (Biederman et al., 1996). Since these families already have dealt with the problems of a girl with AD/HD plus an oppositional defiant disorder, they probably have been exposed to most of the helpful techniques. It is likely that their daughter has already been identified in some way in the system, so that the parents have a network of support.

The AD/HD plus conduct disorder combination is probably one of the most resistant combinations to treatment, and is highly correlated with delinquency, substance abuse, and generally poorer outcomes. It has been shown that those girls with AD/HD who do not manifest hyperactivity are rarely associated with either of these disruptive behavior disorders, which involve impulsive acting-out behaviors. The majority of girls with AD/HD, whether due to lack of hyperactivity or in response to gender-role pressure or both, tend much more toward the internalizing disorders, such as depression or anxiety.

Co-existing developmental disorders

Developmental disorders are another category of potential co-existing disorders which include specific learning disabilities and speech/language disorders. Suspicion of a developmental disorder may require a consultation or assessment by a specialist in these areas, since misdiagnosis often occurs. Many girls who are identified as 'learning disabled' in school turn out to be girls with AD/HD who are underachieving so dramatically that they appear to have specific learning disabilities when they don't. On the other hand, sometimes the underachievement of a girl with AD/HD is complicated by a learning disability in one or more of the following areas: auditory processing, visual processing, sensory integration, memory, motor coordination, or visual-motor integration.

Auditory processing difficulties that may be seen in girls with AD/HD may involve a number of skills, including auditory acuity, discrimination, memory, and synthesis. A parent might begin to suspect auditory processing problems if a daughter has difficulty understanding what is said to her, if she responds inappropriately to what was said, or if she responds very slowly when spoken to. Before exploring an auditory processing problem, a complete hearing test is indicated to rule out any contributing physiological factors.

It is important to remember that slow auditory-processing can reflect the distraction of AD/HD as much as it can a true auditory processing disorder. For this reason, it is critical that the examiner who assesses your daughter's skills not just provide test scores, but also "test the limits" of those abilities. Testing the limits is important in order to clarify whether she has impaired skills relative to other children her age, or whether she has normal skills, but is slowed down for other reasons.

Reading comprehension problems. It is generally agreed that reading acuity and comprehension involve a complex inter-action of numerous variables, including the learner, the prior background knowledge the reader has of the topic, the read-ing strategies, the text material, and concentration. When parents suspect a reading problem, they should first schedule a complete visual exam for their daughter. If a girl with AD/HD demonstrates difficulty with sight word recognition or phon-ics, it may reflect a problem with some aspect of the complex reading ability. In fact, dyslexia often co-occurs with AD/HD. However, many girls with AD/HD find that reading, especially about topics that don't particularly interest them, does not arouse their brains enough to keep them alert. There-fore, they may get distracted and drift off, reread the same sentence repeatedly because they are unable to concentrate on its meaning, hyper focus on the punctuation or print style, or even fall asleep. In all of these cases, the overt problem is that the girl reads or responds slowly; it is then the role of the specialist to dissect the problem and find out why.

Speech and language problems. In general, AD/HD girls are more likely to manifest speech and language problems than are their peers without AD/HD. Often, the developmental history, taken from the parents, reveals that the milestone of the onset of talking was significantly delayed. More than half of all language-based disorders originate from poor attentional control during early development, as well as from a decreased ability to lock language into long-term memory.

Since expressive language problems are far more likely than receptive language problems, it is not surprising that the capacity of a girl with AD/HD to use language overtly or covertly, as a way of guiding her behavior and controlling her impulses may be limited.

Sensory integration problems. When there are sensory integration problems, a child may have trouble translating input from one sensory channel into a response involving another sensory channel. The most common examples involve the visual and auditory realms, such as seeing a letter flash on a computer monitor, and responding to it by pressing a specific key on the keyboard. This type of computerized test often is used to assess distractibility, but a low score can reflect sensory integration difficulties as well. Similarly, forgetting may reflect true memory deficits, or there may be some distraction between taking in the information and retrieving it from memory. While language-based difficulties do respond to remediation, determining if there is a true impairment of skills in addition to the obstacles posed by AD/HD is the first step.

Visual-motor difficulties. Poor handwriting is often a hallmark of AD/HD, but it may also reflect visual-motor difficulties. Similarly, difficulty with jigsaw puzzles or swinging the bat just after the ball crosses the plate, can be signs of visual-motor impairment, or it can suggest divided attention.

Tourette's syndrome. There also is a significant overlap between AD/HD and Tourette's Syndrome, a tic disorder. About 50% of children with Tourette's Syndrome also have AD/HD, and a significant minority of AD/HD children also have a motor or vocal tic. However, this is much more frequently seen in boys (Spencer et al., 1995).

Helping the families of girls with AD/HD

Family counseling is a safe environment in which to explore a wide variety of issues related to AD/HD. Counseling sessions can occur in any family configuration, including parents alone, parents and their daughter, the whole nuclear family, or a parent-child pair, if they are locked in a particular struggle. Some common areas of focus follow.

Processing the diagnosis

Parents need time to understand and accept that their daughter is different and requires special considerations. They may feel relieved by the diagnosis, but overwhelmed by the process of learning how to deal with it. They may feel frustration about past misdiagnoses, and anger at how their child has been treated by the unenlightened in the past. They may experience the stages of a grief reaction, mourning the loss of a "normal" child. They may be fearful about what the future holds for their daughter—and for them. They may feel depressed about the prospect of committing their lives to managing this difficult child. Changing their expectations for their child, and then communicating those new expectations to others, is a stressful and rarely linear process. Parents will stumble through this painful journey at their own rates of speed. For each parent, different aspects of the AD/HD picture will be blind spots. Well-meaning extended family can place additional pressure on a parent. And to make the process even harder, the parents should present a united front to their child.

Understanding how the family system functions

Family counseling is an important intervention designed to help the family unite in the challenge of managing AD/HD. By viewing AD/HD as a stress inducing systemic problem that affects everyone in the household, the family can work to create a more peaceful AD/HD-friendly environment within the home. The therapist helps them to identify underlying family interaction patterns that exacerbate tension and chaos. Through practical problem-solving, the parents are helped to regain their authority and feel in control of the family, perhaps for the first time.

Goals for family interactions must be realistic. Families that cope with AD/HD typically develop a style of communication using high-stimulation language that captures attention, whether it's shouting, slamming a door, crying, threatening to leave, or stamping feet. This style of communication may not change drastically because the AD/HD brain's need for arousal sometimes demands this level of drama and passion. What can change is the content of these communications—it no longer has to be angry, critical or hurtful. A family that can learn to sing the praises of a girl's "islands of competence" will begin to repair damaged self-esteem in a language the girl can understand.

Parent-child communication

Parent-child communication, which likely has been strained to the breaking point, can definitely improve to minimize the frequency and intensity of discord. Once parents begin to understand the diagnosis, they may feel that they always must be understanding and avoid getting angry at their daughter. It is absolutely normal to get angry at one's child from time to time; it doesn't mean the parents don't love her enough, and they shouldn't feel guilty about their anger. Working through these feelings involves separating their feelings about who their daughter really is from feelings about the brain wiring that affects her. Above all, trying to keep a sense of humor about family patterns may help to prevent the escalation of tension that can make family life a constant challenge.

Learning to reframe

Another central aspect of family counseling is to help parents learn to validate their daughter's experience, which is the first step to raising her self-esteem. This can be achieved, in part, by reframing the girl's identity. Reframing does not imply denial or rejection of the problematic aspects of AD/HD; instead, in keeping with a strengths-based assessment, the complex picture can be balanced by focusing on some of the aspects of AD/HD that can be used to one's advantage. This is accomplished by helping the girl and her family to embrace their daughter's unique strengths and aptitudes, and to celebrate the creativity and spontaneity that springs from nonlinear thinking.

Parent support groups

One of the most important results of participating in a parent support group is that parents of AD/HD girls, who are generally quite isolated in their difficulties, can have their experiences validated and normalized. They can obtain detailed and knowledgeable information about behavior management, and can pick up other effective parenting techniques. They also can describe a given dilemma and have the group brainstorm possible solutions. Groups like CHADD (Children and Adults with Attention Deficit Disorder) offer lectures, a lending library of books and videos, and lists of resources. Above all, a family that had been struggling alone in confusion and humiliation can immediately become immersed in a supportive network that can also serve as a safety net.

Overall parenting style has a massive impact on the success of an intervention program: those parents who can anticipate problems, choose their battles wisely, remain calm, are consistent, and communicate acceptance are far more likely to enjoy a collaboration that works for their daughter.

Developing a treatment plan

If you are the parent of a daughter with AD/HD, and you are working with a professional who is knowledgeable and experienced in treating the special needs of girls with AD/HD, you are indeed fortunate. If you have not been so lucky, you face a daunting challenge. Becoming an active advocate for your daughter means educating yourself to the point where you can educate the community about girls with AD/HD in general, and about the very specific needs of your daughter. If you don't live in a metropolitan area or near a major university, you may be a lonely pioneer. While this may not be an easy role, we hope that this book helps you to understand your daughter's needs, to know your rights, and to obtain the supports, accommodations, and professional services that your daughter needs and deserves.

Fortunately, there are parents who have gone before you, working fiercely at times, to create a supportive and consistent AD/HD-friendly environment in which their daughters can thrive. Each of these families served as strong advocates for their daughters. Each, in their unique way, worked to help their daughters find a path that would lead her to recognize and respect her differences, so that she can develop the best of herself. As parents, professionals, and teachers following in the wake of these pioneering efforts, we can benefit from their experience. We each can do our part to extend their efforts to make life in the family, school, and community more accepting of their differences and more appreciative of the talents and abilities of these girls.

Most professionals agree that the only truly successful approach to AD/HD treatment is a comprehensive multi-modal team approach. The collaborative team includes the child, parents, educators, mental health professionals, and medical professionals. A collaborative team is crucial because dueling professionals can serve only to further stress, confuse, and alienate the already struggling family. A comprehensive plan should cover four areas: support and interventions for the whole family, school success, success in community activities, and effective medical treatment.

While diagnosis usually follows the form of the medical model, which focuses on illness and pathology, the treatment plan for an AD/HD girl may be more effective if it stems from a strengths-based assessment. This more holistic perspective acknowledges the problem areas, but creates a treatment plan by building on the strengths of the girl and her family support system. By using the vital and healthy aspects of the family system, the family is empowered to heal itself. While professionals are essential collaborators in the process, the family is able to see that it is within their power to create an AD/HD-friendly environment, custom-tailored to their daughter's needs, that can be workable for all.

The parents' role

In any treatment plan, the role of the parents is paramount. Parents provide information and feedback to the team, observe the child in the widest variety of settings, dispense medications, and implement behavior-management strategies. They advocate for their daughters when their daughters are unable to do so for themselves. And, above all, no part of a treatment plan can be administered without the parents' agreement and participation; without their blessing, any treatment plan is doomed.

The teachers' role

The teacher is responsible for facilitating the school intervention plan that has been developed. They are responsible for implementing both the regular education accommodations and the specialized modifications to maximize learning, academic achievement, and successful behavior management. Teachers also are a valuable source of feedback. They observe your daughter for a significant portion of the day, five days a week. They see how your daughter functions when you, as parents, are not present; sometimes, these reports are surprising. They see the impact of medication, and can give precise information about when the medication seems to kick in, and when it may be wearing off. By being educated and sensitized to your daughter's differences, they will have a basis for interpreting her behaviors and intervening earlier in a difficult situation.

The psychologist's role

The child psychologist can diagnose and assess the disorder

using a combination of checklists, interviews, test instruments, reports from other professionals, and clinical observations. If an assessment of general cognitive functioning is necessary, a psychologist can administer the indicated tests and interpret the data in terms of strengths and weaknesses, as well as clarify the cognitive style of the child. They also consult with teachers concerning educational and behavioral interventions, conduct individual and group therapy as well as skills training, and consult with parents around effective home management issues and emotional issues that may arise. They also assist in day-to-day medication monitoring, and issue-by-issue problem solving. They provide support and encouragement for the daughter and her parents.

The physician's role

The pediatrician rules out other medical explanations for the symptoms, and gets a baseline description of the child's physical status and developmental history before medication is begun. When medication is indicated, a pediatrician or child psychiatrist can prescribe it. When there are co-existing diagnoses that also may require pharmacological intervention, a psychiatrist or other sub-specialist may be the more appropriate professional to join the team.

Examples of customized treatment plans

Many parents have shared descriptions of their daughters with us. We are using four of these descriptions to illustrate some of the many ways that AD/HD can play out at each developmental stage. These four girls had just been seen for an initial consultation, and their overwrought parents asked us, "What's next?"

Amanda, age four, is described by her father:

———— ～～～ ————

"Amanda was active even when she was in her mother's belly—kicking, turning over, hiccuping; it seemed like she never slept. She walked really early, too early, and by 10 months she was running. She never stopped moving, never napped, but would just fall asleep right in the middle of an activity. By the time she was three, she had stitches in her forehead, from falling from the bathroom counter when she was trying to reach the toothbrushes, and in her hand, after she repeatedly pulled on the nose of a neighbor's dog. If you can believe this, she's been 'expelled' from two nursery schools; one couldn't manage her biting and spitting, and one felt that if she couldn't remain seated quietly during circle time, she'd be better off elsewhere.

She absolutely refused to give up her pacifier, and I'm embarrassed to say she still uses it to go to sleep at night. Even so, she's up at least an hour later than she's supposed to be. And then, it's impossible to get her dressed in the morning. We try to get her to dress herself, but we end up fighting with her and doing it ourselves. Sometimes she hugs other kids so hard that they get knocked down and cry. But she's just happy to see them.

During her one-on-one kindergarten readiness screening, they told us that Amanda had some physical coordination problems, both gross motor (she couldn't hop or skip), and fine motor (she pressed so hard on the crayon that it broke in two). They said that all the kids were supposed to run around these orange cones, but each time she ran past one, she grabbed it and took it with her. They said that was

*unusual and that's when we told them she had just
been diagnosed with AD/HD. They recommended that
Amanda start a pre-K program in the fall, and put off
kindergarten another year."*

〰〰

Amanda's treatment plan might include:

- An examination by a developmental pediatrician
  or pediatric neurologist to confirm the AD/HD
  diagnosis, and to rule out other possible causes
  for her behavior.

- A consultation with a child psychologist who
  can evaluate Amanda's cognitive, behavioral,
  and emotional functioning. With that information, the psychologist can help the parents
  develop an appropriate behavior modification
  plan, and provide parent counseling as necessary. The psychologist also can assist the
  parents in finding a preschool setting that can
  accommodate Amanda's needs, and interface
  with the teacher as necessary.

- An evaluation by the Committee on Preschool
  Special Education (CPSE) to determine if
  Amanda meets the criteria for receiving support
  services, such as placement in a therapeutic
  nursery setting, which can offer a very low
  child-teacher ratio, and is well suited for addressing individual needs.

- Amanda's parents should make every effort to
  create a structured and predictable home environment, including firm adherence to a behavior
  modification plan.

- Include a lot of physical exercise in Amanda's daily routine so that she can expend excess energy in a safe and socially acceptable way. Consider enrollment in a Gymboree-type program that targets different muscle groups.

- Amanda's parents should consider joining the local C.H.A.D.D. chapter (Children and Adults with Attention Deficit Disorders), that holds monthly meetings offering parent support, speakers, a lending library of AD/HD materials, and a list of area resources.

Allison, age eight, who has been diagnosed with depression is described by her mother:

"It was never easy to comfort Allison. When she was upset, she'd be like a self-contained unit. She curled up into a ball and sat in the corner. No talking, no crying, just rocking herself. She'd ignore you like you weren't there. She seems unhappy a lot of the time, but she doesn't complain about anything special. I wonder if a girl of eight can be depressed. Allison likes to stay back on the fringes of things, although I guess she'd join a game if someone came up and asked her. Her teacher says she does OK on her work, but she won't speak up in class, and she avoids eye contact.

She still drags around this baby blanket that's in shreds, and sucks on the corner of it. She loves soft things like that; she's only got one pair of pajamas she's willing to wear. She has this one friend across the street who's two years younger, but all they do is play Nintendo. Allison is such a couch potato. One thing, though: she loves to draw, and spends hours in her room with this new set of markers she got for her birthday. When I came in her room and said I really liked her drawings, she looked surprised and said, 'Sometimes, it feels like I'm no good at anything.' That really bothered me, because I used to feel the same way when I was a kid."

Allison's treatment plan might include:

- Teacher implementation of interventions designed by a psychologist to address inattentive symptoms and shyness in the classroom.

- Consult with a psychologist about therapy, which might include cognitive re-framing techniques to improve self-esteem. Because of her genetics and tendency to internalize, Allison should be considered at risk for depression and assessed periodically.

- Schedule a standardized test battery if problems in cognitive functioning are suspected.

- Find a structured extracurricular activity of high interest to Allison that can provide a circumscribed opportunity for peer interaction.

- Focus on one-on-one play dates with a prearranged ending time and parental guidance.

- Consider getting a small furry pet (gerbil, hamster) to help her work through her tactile defensiveness.

► Help her focus on her art as "an island of competence" by offering her art lessons, keeping her supplied with materials, and framing some of her work and hanging it up in the house.

Karen, age 12, who also has AD/HD is described by her mother:

"Karen is so popular! She has shiny dark hair and dark eyes that flash when she smiles. She's always on the phone, giggling with her friends, boys and girls. She's the one to come up with crazy ideas like, "Let's call up each boy in the class, and when they answer, we'll hang up!" But the way she talks, with so much charisma, she gets everyone going. She just loves being the center of attention, and I always say she should be an actress. She gets in trouble for talking in class; last week, she made a nasty comment about the teacher, but the teacher heard it because Karen always talks really loud and fast. But even when she goes to detention, she has fun. She doesn't always remember homework assignments and, when she does, she finishes really quickly so she can get back to her friends. She goes into town every day after school and hangs with a bunch of kids near the pizza place. It drives me nuts that she always comes home late, no matter what I do. Karen just started 'going out' with Mike—he's in 8th grade—so she thinks they are THE cool couple and school's just not that important. What can I do? She's already boy crazy!"

A sample treatment plan for Karen might include:

- Parent training sessions to learn techniques for limit-setting.

- Frank parent-child discussions about safe sex and the risk of pregnancy. Also, be explicit about your values and expectations about smoking, drugs and alcohol.

- AD/HD therapy group to learn/practice self-monitoring skills.

- Regular consultation with teachers, encouraging them to contact you frequently with input.

- Discussion of puberty and its impact on AD/HD symptoms, facilitated by a professional.

- Use of a coach to keep schoolwork on track, and remove mother from that struggle.

- Consult with a psychiatrist for an evaluation for medication.

- Buy a beeper for Karen, so that you can easily contact her wherever she is.

- Link privileges, such as phone and social time, to school performance.

- Consider transfer to private school with more supervision.

- Structure some after school and weekend time.

Lindsay, age 16, is described by her mother:

"Lindsay is a terrific girl, just terrific. She studies hard, and stays up late doing it. And she usually gets good grades. That's how I got through law school. But she worries a lot about school, because she works really slowly. Another problem is that she's a lazy reader; she starts to read and then falls asleep on her book. Lately, she's been losing weight, which was fine at first. It's better to control food than to let it control you, right? But now she seems obsessed with not eating. And all the clothes she buys now are either black or white. She says she doesn't have any big decisions getting dressed in the morning because everything matches now. She must have at least six pairs of black pants, each one in a smaller size than the one before, and they're in size order in the closet. I tell her that organizing her clothes like that takes up a lot of time, but she doesn't seem to care. I don't like to argue with her because when she finally loses it, watch out! She doesn't have a lot of friends, but she has one best friend, Jody. Believe it or not, they love to play Scrabble, but Jody hates it when Lindsay takes forever to put a word down, and instead straightens all the tiles. I would never have thought AD/HD could look like this."

A sample treatment plan for Lindsay might include:

➤ Evaluation for anorexia and other co-existing conditions, such as obsessive-compulsive disorder by a psychiatrist, who can explain the impact of hormonal fluctuations on AD/HD, rule out other explanations for weight loss, and evaluate Lindsay for medication.

☞ Consult with a psychologist about individual treatment.

☞ Find a therapeutic peer support group so that Lindsay can practice socialization skills.

☞ Teach Lindsay self-advocacy skills.

☞ Understand that reading difficulties are common for girls with AD/HD, and not due to laziness; get books on tape.

Clearly, every girl with AD/HD is unique. In fact, there are few disorders that can present with such widely disparate symptoms while having the same underlying neurological picture. Age, temperament, family environment, heredity, interests, and abilities all contribute to the unique experience of each girl with AD/HD. And, in order to maximize each girl's success, her needs require specialized and individualized interventions. In every case, the long-term goal is the same—to help each girl with AD/HD to feel as independent and empowered as possible.

The paths carved out by the girls and their families in this book are examples of possible symptom pictures, and may not be suitable plans for every girl with AD/HD. Our hope is that we have presented varied and flexible models for parents, professionals, and teachers to consider and adapt. Ultimately, it is the goal of that committed team to help these girls reach their fullest potential, with their self-esteem intact, and with pride in the person they are becoming.

Chapter Eleven

Medication—Finding What Works

Medicating girls with AD/HD is often considerably more complicated than medicating boys due to the issues of hormones and the coexisting conditions discussed in Chapter Four. Stimulants, such as methylphenidate (Ritalin) and dextroamphetamine (Dexedrine, Adderall), remain the medications of choice for treating the symptoms of AD/HD. However, in order to address all of the symptoms a girl with AD/HD might be experiencing, unique and therapeutic combinations may need to be considered.

AD/HD and mood disorders

As discussed previously, mood disorders, anxiety, and depression are the most commonly coexisting conditions seen in these girls. While the stimulants increase attention and decrease distractibility, they also may increase anxiety and depression. In addition, obsessive/compulsive traits may be worsened by the stimulants. How, then, is one to handle these combined problems?

Establishing the diagnosis of AD/HD and depression

First, it is critical to establish that AD/HD is the proper diagnosis. In the case of depression, it is important to determine whether the depressive symptoms are secondary to the failure and poor self-esteem associated with the AD/HD, or if there is a true biologic depression in addition to the AD/HD diagnosis.

Treatment with stimulants

Once the diagnosis has been established, treatment usually follows one of two paths. If AD/HD and its aftermath are the cause of the depressed mood, the use of stimulants as part of a multi-modal treatment program should quickly enhance functioning and improve overall well being. Nothing succeeds like success in improving one's mood and overall outlook.

If a girl with AD/HD also has a biologic depression, treatment becomes more complicated. In those cases, the treating physician may elect to prescribe a stimulant and an antidepressant. Side effects and efficacy determine this combination on a case by case basis. Some girls may respond better to one stimulant over another. In each case, optimum response is usually determined by trial and error, with the caveat that if one stimulant does not work, the other should be tried.

Alternatives to stimulants

There are, however, alternative approaches for treating

AD/HD with a concurrent depression. One way is through the use of the class of drugs known as the tricyclic antidepressants (TCAs). These drugs include imipramine, desipramine, and nortriptyline. Studies have shown that this class of drugs addresses both the depressive and AD/HD symptomatology (Pliszka, 1987). They seem to be efficacious in from 60% to 70% of individuals with AD/HD (Huessy and Wright, 1970; Donnelly et al., 1986). Those girls with co-existing mood disorders, depression, or tics may respond better to the TCAs than the stimulants. With these drugs, however, maximum response may not be seen for several weeks, although the symptoms of hyperactivity, anxiety, or mood swings may decrease within a few days. It is important to be aware of this fact and to give these drugs an appropriate trial period before one decides whether or not they are effective. This group of medications also has another drawback in that cardiovascular side effects have been reported in a few cases, and close monitoring of cardiac status with EKG's is necessary during the trial period. These drugs also should not be used in girls with a history of cardiac arrhythmia or a family history of sudden death.

Wellbutrin

Recently, another antidepressant, Wellbutrin, has been introduced for the treatment of both the AD/HD and depressive symptomatology. The few studies that have been done indicate that Wellbutrin may be just as effective as Ritalin for AD/HD symptomatology (Clay et al., 1988; Casat et al., 1989), but it is not without its problems. Wellbutrin is known to lower the seizure threshold and should be used with caution and in low doses for that reason. It can also increase the tics of Tourette's patients, not unlike the stimulants. This medication is mainly being used now in girls after puberty, with warnings regarding changes in menses and libido. While symptoms of depression may be significantly decreased, some girls and women also are reporting that they are more irritable, and suffer cognitive "clouding or confusion" after a period of time on medication.

Clonidine

Stimulants may increase anxiety and, in some girls, the symptoms of depression. In these cases, it is important that the coexisting conditions be treated adequately in addition to the AD/HD. The use of stimulants is not contraindicated, but caution should be exercised. Anti-anxiety medications may be used, but, recently, the use of clonidine has proven quite effective. Clonidine is an alpha2-noradrenergic receptor agonist that has been found to be particularly effective in children who are hyper aroused, over vigilant, and overanxious. It also is effective (about 70% of the time) in treating behavioral symptoms and has been proposed as an alternative to the stimulants.

Selective serotonin re-uptake inhibitors

For girls with true panic attacks, the use of the SSRIs (Selective Serotonin Reuptake Inhibitors) may be quite effective in combination with a stimulant. The SSRI's (Zoloft, Prozac), while effective for treating a variety of disorders including depression, obsessive-compulsive disorders, and panic, are not, in general, indicated for use as a primary drug for the treatment of AD/HD symptoms.

The drug Effexor may be an exception to this statement. Recent information indicates that it is about to be approved as a drug for the treatment of AD/HD.

AD/HD, stimulants, and eating problems

Girls with AD/HD develop unusual and sometimes serious eating problems. It is widely known that stimulants generally decrease appetite. However, for some girls, their inattentiveness and hyperactivity cause them to "forget" about eating, and they tend to eat erratically and to "skip" meals. They also may sit down to a prepared meal and "forget" to eat because they are talking so much and are distracted by all that is going on around them. The food just "sits" on their plates. For these girls, stimulants may help them focus and pay attention to eating. Another group of girls may tend to "binge," and once they begin eating they have difficulty stopping, or they impulsively eat anything in sight, even when they are not hungry. Stimulant medication also may help these girls "stop and think" before eating, or decrease their appetites if they tend to overeat.

Other girls are reported to be "picky" eaters, and have difficulty with food textures. For these girls, stimulant medication may complicate the picture. A "picky" eater on stimulants now also has no appetite. Serving preferred foods and increasing or supplementing caloric intake may be necessary as part of the treatment for this group. For girls who are overweight because of eating too much or not knowing when to stop, this "side effect" can be used to advantage. Under supervision, with a controlled plan, some weight loss may be achieved. A related concern is the girl who abuses medication and its side effects to lose weight. All individuals, male or female, should have regular follow-ups with the prescribing physician, including height and weight checks. Possible side effects should always be discussed, and weight loss issues may need to be addressed, if this seems to be a problem. Additional counseling or referrals to a nutritionist and mental health professional also may be necessary.

AD/HD and PMS

PMS and its associated irritability and mood swings often need to be addressed in the adolescent girl with AD/HD. As stated previously, it appears that many girls with AD/HD suffer from severe PMS symptomatology. Recent studies in the general population indicate that this condition responds to the group of antidepressants in the SSRI category. These include Zoloft, Prozac, and Paxil. Girls with AD/HD, who also experience PMS, may need to be treated with one of these drugs, in addition to their stimulants. The picture becomes even more complicated if a girl has depression, PMS, and AD/HD. Rather than place her on two antidepressants, in addition to her stimulant therapy, it would seem preferable to place her on a SSRI and a stimulant. However, the prescribing physician should be aware that the SSRI dosage might need to be increased prior to menstruation to address the PMS irritability. The maintenance dose of the SSRI used to treat depression effectively may not be enough to treat the PMS symptoms, and managing these symptoms appears to be critical in some girls. Low-dose hormone replacement recently has also been attempted, and seems to aid in evening out mood and decreasing rage and depression in this group.

AD/HD and depression

Co-occurring AD/HD and depression has been discussed above under mood disorders, but because of the great variety of medications available to treat this combination, several treatment regimes will be presented here. Studies looking at combined therapy for children with AD/HD and co-existing conditions indicate that after inadequate response to a methylphenidate alone, treatment with both methylphenidate and fluoxetine reduces depressive symptoms by two-thirds, with global improvement in functioning by about one-third in these children (Gammon & Brown, 1993). The tricyclic antidepressants also may be effective in children with depression or anxiety occurring concomitantly with AD/HD. In studies of children who were non-responders to stimulants, 67% showed marked improvement on the tricyclics (Huessy & Wright, 1970). Wellbutrin is another antidepressant that has been proposed as an alternative to the use of stimulants in children.

Treating AD/HD and bipolar disorder

Children with AD/HD, particularly adolescent girls and young women, are now being more frequently diagnosed with bipolar disorder, in addition to their AD/HD. In these cases, it is important to be sure to differentiate the diagnosis of bipolar disorder from AD/HD and depression, which tends to be seen more commonly in females. While AD/HD and bipolar disorder can co-occur, it is usually the AD/HD that is diagnosed first. However, once the diagnosis of bipolar disorder is made, by a professional well-trained in differentiating the symptoms of AD/HD from mania and hypo-mania, it is imperative to treat both the bipolar disorder and the AD/HD to assure improvement. Lithium, or the anticonvulsant, Depakote, is usually prescribed as the treatment of choice for the bipolar disorder for a period of five to ten days alone to address the bipolar symptoms. After that period, a stimulant may be added to effectively treat the AD/HD symptomatology, without the danger of increasing the cycling of the bipolar disorder which can occur when treatment is undertaken with stimulants alone. Concurrent treatment for both of these conditions is imperative, and prognosis for improvement is poor if either condition remains untreated.

Brianna's story—a complex treatment case study

Brianna was a beautiful, tall, dark-haired, 15-year old when she was referred, during her first year in high school, for evaluation of possible attention deficit disorder. At that time, Brianna reported that she had a great deal of difficulty sitting still and concentrating. She was distracted easily by both visual and auditory stimuli. Some impulsive behaviors were noted, and Brianna was known for her constant talking. Visual images and doodling would help focus Brianna during lectures, and she frequently used an outline to stay on track. She was poor at note-taking and doodled rather than taking notes in class. Brianna reported that she was a slow reader and did not like to read.

In addition to these problems, Brianna had an overly developed awareness of germs. She constantly felt that she must wash her hands, and that others must wash their hands before touching her or her things. She also reported that she felt "unbalanced" if her body was touched. There was a need to have everything symmetrical. If she was touched on one side, she then must touch the other side in order to feel better.

Brianna had had seizures as a newborn until nine

months of age. As a small child, she was hypersensitive to touch and textures. As a preschooler, Brianna was described as being hyperactive, messy, and having difficulty with transitions. It had always been difficult for her to fall asleep at night, and she had given up her naps early. Her family history included other family members diagnosed with tics, OCD, and auditory processing problems.

Upon completion of neurodevelopmental and educational assessments, including reports from her parents and teachers, Brianna was diagnosed as having attention deficit/hyperactivity disorder (AD/HD) and obsessive compulsive disorder (OCD). Primary recommendations were for a trial of stimulant medication and counseling. Tutoring was also undertaken to improve organizational, note taking, and reading comprehension skills. It was explained to Brianna that the stimulant medication, while alleviating her difficulty with concentrating and her hyperactivity, could possibly complicate her OCD symptoms or tics.

Brianna decided that her AD/HD symptoms were the most prevalent and bothersome, and the ones that she elected to treat. Alternative and additional medication interventions were also discussed at that time.

Brianna was placed on methylphenidate, and close monitoring was undertaken. Brianna and her teachers reported positive changes at school. Her germ phobia was perceived as being a little worse, or, perhaps, she was more aware of it. At home, her parents noted increased irritability and slight appetite decrease. She continued on this regime for approximately a year. At that time, Brianna reported that her OCD was getting worse and that she was more irritable and jittery. She decided that she would like to try medication to address these problems as well. She began a trial of clonidine and experienced a significant reduction in phobias, irritability, and OCD symptoms.

Over the next year, however, Brianna developed full-blown panic attacks. She began taking Prozac and used relaxation and biofeedback techniques. When her clonidine was discontinued, her OCD symptoms returned. AD/HD symptoms remained under control with methylphenidate, but her grades were inconsistent because of an inability to sustain effort at times. Panic attacks abated over the next two months. The stimulant and SSRI combination was maintained for another year. At that time, the SSRI was decreased to every other day and eventually was taken only for the week before her period.

Brianna began college that next fall with accommodations for her AD/HD and OCD symptoms and continued to do well on her stimulant medication. She required a single dorm room, preferential registration to allow her to arrange her class schedule so that she could schedule classes when her medications were maximally effective, extended time on tests because of her slow reading rate and need to re-read, and note-takers for lecture classes.

Brianna's case seems typical for many girls with AD/HD who manifest anxiety-related disorders in addition to their AD/HD, and illustrates the necessity to treat each symptom complex in order to effectively improve overall functioning. Brianna was at times immobilized by her OCD or panic/anxiety, which worsened after puberty. However, with appropriate treatment, Brianna had stabilized by college, and she could manage her symptoms effectively with a little additional support.

Conclusion

Diagnosing AD/HD is not a simple matter, under the best of circumstances. Include co-existing conditions and gender issues and you add layers of complexity to this process. In addition, physiological factors may have a significant impact, not only on the diagnosis, but also on the choice of treatment regimes and outcomes. Professionals involved in the diagnostic process need to be made aware of the additional burdens a girl may be carrying. Societal and hormonal stressors need to be assessed and addressed in treatment. The use of medication in girls with AD/HD may not be as simplistic as the choice of a stimulant, but may involve a more sophisticated approach, using combination therapies and/or hormone replacement. Educators, mental health professionals, physicians, parents, and the girls themselves need to be made more aware and become more knowledgeable about the unique presentation of AD/HD in girls. Through increased knowledge, understanding will follow. And it is only with increased understanding that improved outcomes will be experienced.

Chapter Twelve

Putting Our Understanding into Action

A s with all ground-breaking topics in the study of human behavior, clinical practice often precedes research. What we offer here is based on the many years of clinical experience that have formed our understanding of girls with AD/HD, and how they can be helped. We hope that our insights and observations lead to much-needed research on girls with AD/HD.

To date, the little research that has been undertaken has been fairly narrowly focused, selecting girls who meet the diagnostic guidelines laid out in the Diagnostic and Statistical Manuals, and comparing them to boys in terms of the classic, male-based criteria of hyperactivity, impulsivity, and distractibility. While this is certainly a necessary first step toward understanding girls, our hope is that research will broaden over time to include more research on gender differences. An essential diagnostic question asks how we can develop and standardize gender appropriate criteria that can take more subtle and internalized symptom patterns into account. We also hope that as the typical issues for girls are better defined, research can focus on treatment modalities that best suit girls. Today, most treatment programs for children with AD/HD focus on problematic behaviors of boys, and how to better control them in the classroom and at home. As we learn more about how to diagnose and treat girls, we hope that programs develop that can help girls with the self-esteem issues and social interaction issues that are so challenging and painful for them.

The earlier we learn to appropriately identify girls with AD/HD, the less potential damage they will suffer. Today, grown women are more likely to be diagnosed than young girls. A likely explanation for this difference in sex ratios found between children and adults is that women have the opportunity for self-referral, whereas girls must rely on parents and teachers to refer them. These women have waited half a lifetime for a diagnosis that can lead to understanding, self-acceptance, and success.

Because greater AD/HD challenges for girls typically develop at puberty, perhaps the next wave of identification will take place in middle and high school. And, as the standard questionnaires used by teachers, parents, and pediatricians to identify young children are appropriately altered to include more female AD/HD patterns, the wave will move down to elementary school-aged girls and to preschoolers. Those who are reading this book today will form the vanguard of parents and professionals that can bring about this new wave of recognition and identification.

Early identification can help both parents, teachers, and other professionals create environments to support and sustain these girls from their earliest years, helping them to feel strong, competent, and aware of their abilities. The more we learn, the more we are aware that the key to helping individuals with AD/HD is to create, or to help them create, a learning and working environment that suits their strengths.

As we emphasized when discussing treatment plans in Chapter Ten, each girl with AD/HD is unique. Those girls who are fortunate enough to be identified very early in life could have the benefit of understanding and supportive parents who make appropriate choices for schooling, playmates, and play activities for their daughters. What a difference it would make:

- If active, outgoing girls with AD/HD had the good fortune to attend preschools that offered them more opportunity for movement, climbing and socializing in action settings.

- If girls who are quiet, disorganized daydreamers had the luxury of small group interaction and more individual attention from teachers.

- If creative girls with AD/HD received more encouragement and validation for their artistic abilities and less discouragement for messiness.

- If girls who are outspoken risk-takers were encouraged in sports or entrepreneurial activities rather than admonished for not being more lady-like.

While many boys with AD/HD need help in controlling their impulses, reducing aggression, and becoming more compliant, many girls with AD/HD need just the opposite! Our daydreaming daughters don't need help in learning to sit down and be quiet; they need lessons in how to stand up and be heard! They need to overcome their fears of asking for help, of raising their hand, of answering the teacher's question. More talkative, outgoing girls with AD/HD need positive outlets for their social energy—permission and encouragement to take leadership positions in the classroom, to use their energy to plan and organize rather than to chatter disruptively. While many classroom guides for teachers emphasize the needs of boys with AD/HD to move about, there is almost no recognition that girls, whose hyperactivity is often verbal, need appropriate, constructive verbal outlets!

For many girls, their struggle is hidden—behind intense efforts to avoid notice, to please the teacher, and to get their work done. The brighter they are, the more easily they can hide their attentional difficulties by compensating with other strengths. Parents and professionals alike must be aware that young girls may successfully avoid overt difficulties for many years. The DSM-IV "requirement" that AD/HD be evident before the age of seven may need to be amended to take these patterns into account. The fact that they were quiet, obedient and above-average students makes their burgeoning AD/HD no less real when it rears its head at puberty.

We are at a very early point on the learning curve in understanding girls with AD/HD. We hope that parents who read this book will share it with professionals and teachers. Teachers should share it with counselors and school psychologists. AD/HD organizations need to sponsor more discussions and presentations on girls with AD/HD. We all need to work together to raise the awareness of parents and professionals so that this generation of girls doesn't have to wait until they are women to finally understand their differences and embrace their strengths.

REFERENCES

Adams, W. (1982). Effect of methylphenidate on thought processing time in children. *Journal of Developmental and Behavioral Pediatrics, 3,* 133-135.

Adesman, A.R.A., Altshuler, L. A., Lipkin, P.H. & Walco, G.A. (1990). Otitis media in children with learning disabilities and in children with attention deficit disorder with hyperactivity. *Pediatrics, 85,* 442-446.

American Psychiatric Association. (1968). *Diagnostic and statistical manual of mental disorders (2nd ed.).* Washington,DC: Author.

American Psychiatric Association. (1980). *Diagnostic and statistical manual of mental disorders (3rd ed.).* Washington, DC: Author.

American Psychiatric Association. (1987). *Diagnostic and statistical manual of mental Disorders (3rd ed., rev.).* Washington, DC: Author.

American Psychiatric Association. (1994). *Diagnostic and statistical manual of mental disorders (4th ed.).* Washington, DC: Author.

Anastopoulos, A. D., DuPaul, G. J., & Barkley, R. A. (1991). Stimulant medication and parent training therapies for attention deficit-hyperactivity disorder. *Journal of Learning Disabilities, 24,* 210-218.

Anderson, S.L., Rutstein, M., Benzo, J.M., et al. (1997). Sex differences in dopamine receptor overproduction and elimination. *NeuroReport, 8,* 1495-1498.

Arcia, E. & Conners, C.K. (1998). Gender Differences in ADHD? *Journal of Developmental and Behavoral Pediatrics, 19,* 77-83.

Arnold, L. E. (1996). Sex differences in ADHD: Conference Summary. *Journal of Abnormal Child Psychology, 24,* 555-568.

Baren, M. (1994). Managing ADHD. *Contemporary Pediatrics, 11,* 29-48.

Barkley, R. A. (1988). The effects of methylphenidate on the interactions of preschool ADHD children with their mothers. *Journal of the American Academy of Child and Adolescent Psychiatry, 27,* 336-341.

Barkley, R. A. (1991). *Attention-Deficit Hyperactivity Disorder: A clinical workbook.* New York: Guilford Press.

Barkley, R. A. (1997). *ADHD and the nature of self-control.* New York: Guilford Press.

Barkley, R. A., Anastopoulos, A. D., Guevremont, D. G., & Fletcher, K. F. (1992). Mother-adolescent interactions, family beliefs and conflicts, and maternal psychopathology. *Journal of Abnormal Child Psychology, 20,* 263-288.

Barkley, R. A., & Cunningham, C. E. (1979). The effects of methylphenidate on the mother-child interactions of hyperactive children. *Archives of General Psychiatry, 36,* 201-208.

Barkley, R. A., DuPaul, G. J., & McMurray, M. B. (1991). Attention deficit disorder with and without hyperactivity: Clinical response to three dose levels methylphenidate. *Pediatrics, 87,* 519-531.

Barkley, R. A., McMurray, M. B., Edelbrock, C. S., & Robbins, K. (1989). The response of aggressive and nonaggressive ADHD children to two doses of methylphenidate. *Journal of the American Academy of Child and Adolescent Psychiatry, 28,* 873-881.

Barkley, R. A., McMurray, M. B., Edelbrock, C. S., & Robbins, K. (1990). Side effects of methylphenidate in children with attention deficit hyperactivity disorder: A systemic, placebo-controlled evaluation. *Pediatrics, 86,* 184-192.

Battle, E. S., & Lacey, B. (1972). A context for hyperactivity in children over time. *Child Development, 43,* 757-773.

Beck, N., Warnke, A., Kruger, H. P., & Barglik, W. (1996). Hyperkinetic syndrome and behavioral disorders in street traffic: A case control pilot study. *Klinik und Poliklinik fur Kinder und Jugendpsychiatrie, 24,* 82-91.

Behar, L., & Stringfield, S. (1974). A behavior rating scale for the preschool child. *Developmental Psychology, 10,* 601-610.

Bell, R. Q., Waldrop, M. F., & Weller, G. M. (1972). A rating system for the assessment of hyperactive and withdrawn children in preschool samples. *American Journal of Orthopsychiatry, 42,* 23-34.

Berry, C. A., Shaywitz, S. E., & Shaywitz, B. A. (1985) Girls with Attention Deficit Disorder: A silent minority? A report on behavioral and cognitive characteristics. *Pediatrics, 76,* 801-809.

Biederman, J., Faraone, S., Mick, E., Williamson, S., Wilens, T., Spencer, T., Weber, W., Jetton, J., Kraus, I., Pert, J., & Zallen, B. (1999). Clinical correlates of AD/HD in females: Findings from a large group of girls ascertained from pediatric and psychiatric referral services. *Journal of the American Academy of Child and Adolescent Psychiatry, 38,* 966-975.

Biederman, J., Faraone, S.V., Keenan, K., et al. (1992). Further evidence for family-genetic risk factors in attention deficit hyperactivity disorder (ADHD): Patterns of comorbidity in probands and relatives in psychiatrically and pediatrically referred samples. *Archives of General Psychiatry, 49,* 728-738.

Biederman, J., Faraone, S. V., Milberger, S., Garcia-Jetton, J., Chen, L., Mick, E., Greene, R., & Russell, R. (1996). Is childhood oppositional defiant disorder a precursor to adolescent conduct disorder? Findings from a four year follow-up study of children with AD/HD. *Journal of the American Academy of Child and Adolescent Psychiatry, 35,* 1193-1204.

Biederman, J., Gastfriend, D. R., & Jellinek, M. S. (1986). Desipramine in the treatment of children with attention deficit disorder. *Journal of Clinical Psychopharmacology, 6,* 359-363.

Biederman, J., Mick, E., & Faraone, S. (1998). Depression in Attention Deficit Hyperactivity Disorder (ADHD) in children: "True" depression or demoralization? *Journal of Affective Disorders, 47,* 113-122.

Biederman J., Milberger, S., Faraone, S., Kiely, K., Guite, J., Mick, E., Ablon, S., Warburton, R., & Reed, E. (1995). Family-environment risk factors for attention-deficit hyperactivity disorder. *Archives of General Psychiatry, 52,* 464-470.

Biederman, J., Newcorn, J., & Sprich, S. (1991). Comorbidity of ADHD with conduct, depressive, anxiety, and other disorders. *American Journal of Psychiatry, 148,* 564-577.

Biederman, J., Santangelo, S.L., Faraone, S.V., Kiely, K., Guite, J., Mick, E., Reed, E.D., Kraus, I., Jellinke, J. & Perrin, J. (1995). Clinical correlates of enuresis in ADHD and non-ADHD children. *Journal of Child Psychology and Psychiatry, 36,* 865-877.

Brown, R.T., Madan-Swain, A., & Baldwin, K. (1991). Gender differences in a clinic-referred sample of attention deficit disordered children. *Child Psychiatry and Human Development, 22,* 111-128.

Brown, R.T., Abramowitz, A. J., Madan-Swain, A., Eckstrand, D., &
Dulcan, M. (1989). *AD/HD gender differences in a clinic
referred sample*. Paper presented at the Annual Meeting of the
American Academy of Child and Adolescent Psychiatry, New
York.

Brown, R.T., & Sexson, S. B. (1988). A controlled trial of methylpheni
date in black adolescents. *Clinical Pediatrics, 27,* 74-81.

Brown, T. E. (1996). Brown Attention Deficit Disorder Scales. San
Antonio, TX: The Psychological Corporation.

Brown, T. E. (1998). *AD/HD in Persons with Superior IQ's:Unique Risks.*
Presented at the 10th Annual CHADD Conference, New York.

Bruun, R. D., Cohen, D. J., & Leckman, J. F. (1989). *Guide to the
diagnosis and treatment of Tourette's Syndrome*. Bayside, NY:
Tourette Syndrome Association.

Bussing, R., Zima, B., Perwien, A., et al. (1998). Children in special
education programs: AD/HD use of services and unmet needs.
American Journal of Public Health, 88, 880-886.

Carlson, C. L., Tamm, L., & Gaub, M. (1996). Gender differences in
children with ADHD, ODD, and co-occurring ADHD/ODD
identified in a school population. *Journal of the American
Academy of Child and Adolescent Psychiatry, 36,* 1706-1714.

Casat, C. D., Pleasants, D. Z., & Schroeder, D. H. (1989). Bupropion in
children with attention deficit disorder. *Psychopharmacology
Bulletin, 25,* 198-201.

Castellanos, F. X., Giedd, J., Marsh, W. L., et al. (1996). Quantitative brain
magnetic resonance imaging in attention-deficit hyperactivity
disorder. *Archives of General Psychiatry, 53,* 607-616.

Caviness, V. S., Kennedy, D. N., Richelme, C., et al. (1996). The human
brain age 7-11 years: A volumetric analysis based on magnetic
resonance images. *Cerebral Cortex, 6,* 726-36.

Chervin, R. D., Dillon, J. E., Bassetti, C., Ganoczy, D. A., & Pituch, K. J.
(1997). Symptoms of sleep disorders, inattention, and hyperactivity in children. *Sleep, 20,* 1185-1192.

Clay, T. H., Gaultieri, C. T., & Evans, R. W. (1988). Clinical and neuropsychological effects of the novel antidepressant bupropion.
Psychopharmacology Bulletin, 24, 143-148.

Coleman, J., Wolkind, S., & Ashley, L. (1977). Symptoms of behavior disturbance and adjustment to school. *Journal of Child Psychology and Psychiatry, 18,* 201-209.

Conners, C. K. (1997). *Conners Teacher Rating Scale – Revised (L).* North Tonawanda, NY: Multi-Health Systems, Inc.

Corkum, P., Tannock, R., & Moldofsky, H. (1998). Sleep disturbances in children with attention-deficit/hyperactivity disorder. *Journal of the American Academy of Child and Adolescent Psychiatry, 37,* 637-646.

Denkla, M. V. (1989). Executive function, the overlap zone between attention deficit hyperactivity disorder and learning disabilities. *International Pediatrics, 4,* 155-160.

Donnelly, M., Zametkin, A. J., Rapoport, J. L., et al. (1986). Treatment of childhood hyperactivity with desipramine: Plasma drug concentration, cardiovascular effects, plasma and urinary catecholamine levels, and clinical response. *Clinical Pharmacology and Therapeutics, 39,* 72-81.

Dorn, L. D., Hitt, S. F., & Rotenstein, D. (1999). Biopsychological and cognitive differences in children with premature vs. on-time adrenarche. *Archives of Pediatric and Adolescent Medicine, 153,* 137-146.

Dulcan, M. K. (1990). Using psychostimulants to treat behavioral disorders of children and adolescents. *Journal of Child and Adolescent Psychopharmacology, 1,* 7-20.

DuPaul, G. J., & Rapport, M. D. (1993). Does methylphenidate normalize the classroom performance of children with attention deficit disorder? *Journal of the American Academy of Child and Adolescent Psychiatry, 32,* 190-198.

Dworkin, P. H., & Levine, M. D. (1980). The preschool child: prediction and prescription. In A.P. Scheiner, & I.F. Abrams, (Eds.), *The practical management of the developmentally disabled child.* St. Louis, MO: Mosby.

Epstein, M. A., Shaywitz, B. A., Shaywitz, J. L., & Woolston, J. L. (1991). Boundaries of attention deficit disorder. *Journal of Learning Disabilities, 24,* 78-86.

Erikson, E. H. (1963). *Childhood and Society (2nd Ed).* New York: W.W. Norton.

Ernst, M., Liebenauer, L. I., King, A., et al. (1994). Reduced brain metabolism in hyperactive girls. *Journal of the American Academy of Child and Adolescent Psychiatry, 33,* 858-868.

Famularo, R., & Fenton, T. (1987). The effect of methylphenidate on school grades in children with attention deficit disorder without hyperactivity: A preliminary report. *Journal of Clinical Psychiatry, 48,* 112-114.

Feldman, H., Crumrine, P., Handen, B. L., et al. (1989). Methylphenidate in children with seizures and attention-deficit disorder. *American Journal of Diseases in Children, 143,* 1081-1086.

Filipek, P. A., Semrud-Clikeman, M., Steingard, R. J., et al. (1997). Volumetric MRI analysis comparing subjects having attention deficit hyperactivity disorder with normal controls. *Neurology, 48,* 589-601.

Fink, G., Sumner, B. E., Rosie, R., Grace, O., & Quinn, J. P. (1996). Estrogen control of central neurotransmission: Effect on mood, mental state, and memory. *Cell Molecular Biology, 16,* 325-344.

Funk, J. B., Chessare, J. B., Weaver, M. T., & Exley, A. R. (1993). Attention deficit hyperactivity disorder, creativity, and the effects of methylphenidate. *Pediatrics, 91,* 816-819.

Gammon, G. D., & Brown, T. E. (1993). Fluoxetine and methylphenidate in combination for treatment of attention deficit disorder and comorbid depressive disorder. *Journal of Child and Adolescent Psychopharmacology, 3,* 1-10.

Gaub, J., & Carlson, C. (1997). Gender differences in AD/HD: A meta-analysis and critical review. *Journal of the American Academy of Child and Adolescent Psychiatry, 36,* 1036-1045.

Gilligan, C. (1982). *In a Different Voice.* Cambridge, MA: Harvard University Press.

Golden, G. S. (1988). The relationship between stimulant medication and tics. *Pediatric Annals, 17,* 405-408.

Goldstein, S. (1993). Young children at risk: Recognizing the early signs of ADHD. *The AD/HD Report, 1(4).* New York: Guilford Press.

Goldstein, S., & Goldstein, M. (1990). *Managing Attention Disorders in children: A guide for practitioners.* New York: John Wiley.

Gredler, G. R. (1984). Transition classes: A viable alternative for the at-risk child? *Psychology in the Schools, 21,* 463- 470.

Grossman, H., & Grossman, S. (1994). *Gender issues in education.* Needham Heights, MA: Allyn & Bacon.

Hartmann, Thom. (1998). Private communication.

Holloway, L. (1999). Holding moonbeams: Developing a group for teen girls with AD/HD. *ADDvance,* 2(6), 12-14. Silver Spring, MD: Advantage Books.

Huessy, H. R. (1990). *The pharmacotherapy of personality disorders in women.* Paper presented at the Annual Meeting of the American Psychiatric Association (symposia), New York.

Huessy, H. R., & Wright, A. L. (1970). The use of imipramine in children's behavior disorders. *International Journal of Child Psychology, 37,* 194-199.

Hunt, R. D., Capper, L., & O'Connell, P. (1990). Clonidine in child and adolescent psychiatry. *Journal of Child and Adolescent Psychopharmacology, 1,* 87-102.

Hunt, R. D., Mindera, R. B., & Cohen, D. J. (1985). Clonidine benefits children with attention deficit disorder and hyperactivity: Report of a double-blind placebo-crossover therapeutic trial. *Journal of the American Academy of Child Psychiatry, 24,* 617-629.

Hynd, G., Semrud-Clikeman, M., Lorys, A. R., Novey, D., & Eliopulos, D., (1990). Brain morphology in developmental dyslexia and attention deficit hyperactivity disorder. *Archives of Neurology, 47,* 919-926.

Hynd, G., Semrud-Clikeman, M., Lorys, A. R., Novey, D., Eliopulos, D., & Lyytinen, H. (1991). Corpus callosum morphology in attention deficit hyperactivity disorder: Morphometric analysis of MRI. *Journal of Learning Disabilities, 24,* 141-146.

Ialongo, N. S., Horn, W. F., Pascoe, J. M., et al. (1993). The effects of a multimodal intervention with attention-deficit hyperactivity disorder children: A 9-month follow-up. *Journal of the American Academy of Child and Adolescent Psychiatry, 32,* 182-189.

Johnson, J., McCown, W., & Booker, M. (1986). *MMPI profiles of multiply abused and sheltered women.* Paper presented at the Annual Meeting of the Midwestern Psychological Association, Chicago.

Jones, C. B. (1989). *Teachers' corner. Kids getting you down?* San Diego: Learning Development Services.

Jones, C. B. (1993). The young and the restless: Helping the preschool child with attention deficit/hyperactivity disorder. *CHADDER.* Plantation, Florida: CHADD.

Keith, R. W., & Engineer, P. (1991). Effects of methylphenidate on the auditory processing abilities of children with attention deficit-hyperactivity disorder. *Journal of Learning Disabilities, 24,* 630-636.

Kinsbourne, M. (1992). Quality of life in children with ADHD. *Challenge, 6,* 1-2.

Lahey, B., & Carlson, C. (1991). Validity of the diagnostic category of attention deficit disorder without hyperactivity: A review of the literature. *Journal of Learning Disabilities, 24,* 110-114.

Liu, C., Robin, A. L., Brenner, S., & Eastman, J. (1991). Social acceptability of methylphenidate and behavior modification for treating attention deficit hyperactivity disorder. *Pediatrics, 88,* 560-565.

Mash, E. J., & Johnson, C. (1982). A comparison of the mother-child interactions of younger and older hyperactive and normal children. *Child Development, 53,* 1371-1381.

Matheny, A. P., Brown, A. M., & Wilson, R. S. (1971). Behavioral antecedents of accidental injuries in early childhood: A study of twins. *Journal of Pediatrics, 79,* 122-124.

Matheny, A. P., Brown, A. M., & Wilson, R. S. (1972). Assessment of children's behavioral characteristics: A tool in accident prevention. *Clinical Pediatrics, 11,* 437-439.

McBridge, M. C., Wang, D. D., & Torres, C. F. (1986). Methylphenidate in therapeutic doses does not lower seizure threshold. *Annals of Neurology, 20,* 428.

McCarney, S. B. (1995). *The Early Childhood Attention Deficit Disorders Evaluation Scale.* Columbia, MO: Hawthorn Educational Services.

McCarney, S. B., & Johnson, N. (1995). *The Early Childhood Attention Deficit Disorders Intervention Manual.* Columbia, MO: Hawthorne Educational Services.

Johnson, J., McCown, W., & Booker, M. (April,1986). *MMPI profiles of multiply abused and sheltered women.* Paper presented at the Meeting of the Midwestern Psychological Association, Chicago, Illinois.

Jones, C. B. (1989). Teachers' corner. *Kids getting you down?* San Diego: Learning Development Services.

Jones, C. B. (1993). The young and the restless: Helping the preschool child with attention deficit/hyperactivity disorder. *CHADDER.* Plantation, Florida: Ch.A.D.D.

Keith, R. W., & Engineer, P. (1991). Effects of methylphenidate on the auditory processing abilities of children with attention deficit-hyperactivity disorder. *Journal of Learning Disabilities*, 24, 630-636.

Kinsbourne, M. (1992). Quality of life in children with ADHD. *Challenge*, 6,1-2.

Lahey, B & Carlson, C. (1991). Validity of the diagnostic category of attention deficit disorder without hyperactivity: A Review of the Literature. *Journal of Learning Disabilities,* 24, 110-114.

Liu, C., Robin, A. L., Brenner, S., & Eastman, J. (1991). Social acceptability of methylphenidate and behavior modification for treating attention deficit hyperactivity disorder. *Pediatrics,* 88, 560-565.

Mash, E. J., & Johnson, C. (1982). A comparison of the mother-child interactions of younger and older hyperactive and normal children. *Child Development*, 53, 1371-1381.

Matheny, A. P., Brown, A. M., & Wilson, R. S. (1971). Behavioral antecedents of accidental injuries in early childhood: A study of twins. *Journal of Pediatrics*, 79, 122-124.

Matheny, A. P., Brown, A. M., & Wilson, R. S. (1972). Assessment of children's behavioral characteristics: A tool in accident prevention. *Clinical Pediatrics*, 11, 437-439.

Quinn, P. O. (1990). If your child is ...,then... In B. Lyons, & M. Janes (Eds.), *Choosing the right school for your child: A guide to selected elementary schools in the Washington area.* (pp. 13-15). Lanham, MD: Madison Books.

Ratey, J. J., Greenberg, M. S., & Lindem, K. J. (1991). Combination of treatments for attention deficit hyperactivity disorder in adults. *The Journal of Nervous and Mental Disease, 179,* 699-701.

Richman, N, Stevenson, J. E., & Graham, P. J. (1975). Prevalence of behavior problems in 3-year-old children: An epidemiological study in a London borough. *Journal of Child Psychology and Psychiatry, 16,* 277-287.

Richardson, W. (1997). *The link between A.D.D. & addiction: Getting the help you deserve.* Colorado Springs, CO: Pinon Press.

Rucklidge, J., & Kaplan, B. (1998). Being identified with ADHD in adult hood: Mental health implications for women. *ADDvance, 2 (2),* 22-28. Silver Spring, MD: Advantage Books.

Ryan, N. D. (1990). Heterocyclic antidepressants in children and adolescents. *Journal of Child and Adolescent Psychopharmacology, 1,* 21-31.

Sallee, F., Stiller, R., Perel, J., & Everett, G. (1989). Pemoline-induced abnormal involuntary movements. *Journal of Clinical Psychopharmacology, 9,* 125-129.

Schleifer, M., Weiss, G., Cohen, N., et al., (1975). Hyperactivity in preschoolers and the effect of methylphenidate. *American Journal of Orthopsychiatry, 45,* 38-50.

Seidman, L. J., Biederman, J., Faraone, S., et al. (1997). A pilot study of neuropsychological function in ADHD girls. *Journal of the American Academy of Child and Adolescent Psychiatry, 36,* 366-373.

Solden, S. (1995). *Women with Attention Deficit Disorder.* Grass Valley, CA: Underwood Books.

Spencer, T., Biederman, J., Harding, M., Wilens, T., & Faraone, S. (1995). The relationship between tic disorders and Tourette's Syndrome revisited. *Journal of the American Academy of Child and Adolescent Psychiatry, 34,* 1133-1139.

Still, G. F. (1902). Some abnormal psychical conditions in children. *Lancet,* *1,* 1008-1012, 1077-1082, 1163-1168.

Swanson, J. M., Cantwell, D., Lerner, M., et al. (1991). Effects of stimulant medication on learning in children with ADHD. *Journal of Learning Disabilities, 24,* 219-230.

Szatmari, P., Offord, D. R., & Boyle, M. H. (1989). Ontario Child Health Study: Prevalence of attention deficit disorder with hyperactivity. *Journal of Child Psychology and Psychiatry, 30,* 219-230.

Tirosh, E., Sadeh, A., Munvez, R., & Lavie, P. (1993). Effects of methylphenidate on sleep in children with attention-deficit hyperactivity disorder. *American Journal of Diseases in Children, 147,* 1313-1315.

Tzelepis, A. (1999). Personal communication.

Vygotsky, L. S. (1978). *Mind in society.* Cambridge, MA: Harvard University Press.

Waldrop, M., Bell, R., McLaughlin, B., & Halverson, C.F. (1978). Newborn minor physical anomalies predict short attention span, peer aggression, and impulsivity at age 3. *Science, 199,* 563-565.

Walker, C. (1999). *Gender and genetics in ADHD: Genetics matter; gender does not.* Paper presented at the ADDA Regional Conference, Chicago.

Wheeler, J., & Carlson, C. (1994). The social functioning of children with ADD with and without hyperactivity: A comparison of their peer relations and social deficits. *Journal of Emotional and Behavioral Disorders, 2,* 2-12.

Whitehouse, D., Shah, U., & Palmer, F. B. (1980). Comparison of sustained-release and standard methylphenidate in the treatment of minimal brain dysfunction. *Journal of Clinical Psychiatry, 41,* 282-285.

Wilens, T. E., & Biederman, J. (1992). The stimulants. *Pediatric Psycopharmacology, 15,* 191-222.

Wilens, T. E., Biederman J., & Spencer, T. (1996). Attention deficit hyperactivity disorders and the psychoactive substance use disorders. In S. Jaffee, (Ed.), *Pediatric substance use disorders* (pp.73-91). Philadelphia: Saunders.

Willerman, L., & Plomin, R. (1973). Activity level in children and their parents. *Child Development, 44,* 854-858.

Zametkin, A. J., Nordahl, T. E., & Gross, M. (1990). Cerebral glucose metabolism in adults with hyperactivity of childhood onset. *New England Journal of Medicine, 323,* 1413-1415.

Index

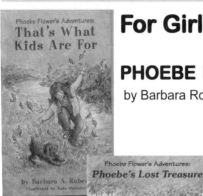

For more information on women and girls with AD/HD

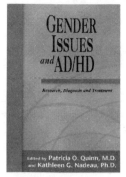

GENDER ISSUES and AD/HD

Research, Diagnosis and Treatment

Edited by Patricia O. Quinn, M.D.
and Kathleen G. Nadeau, Ph.D.

ISBN: 0-9714609-1-4
$39.00   468 pages

Gender Issues and AD/HD:
Research, Diagnosis and Treatment
edited by Patricia Quinn, M.D. and Kathleen Nadeau, Ph.D.

Finally! An in-depth resource on gender issues and AD/HD covering topics that have received little attention elsewhere including the need to rethink DSM-IV diagnostic criteria, the impact of hormones on AD/HD in women, the use of medications during pregnancy, and the range of coexisting conditions that complicate and often mask AD/HD in females. A self-report inventory for women is introduced as a tool to help clinicians consider important gender related issues during the diagnostic process.

Understanding Women with AD/HD

edited by Kathleen Nadeau, Ph.D. and Patricia Quinn, M.D.

Understanding Women is designed to be a practical and readable guide for women at any age. Chapters focus on different stages of life and address life's challenges including motherhood, romance, the single life, sexuality, getting organized, and taking charge. If you are a women with AD/HD, this is the book that can help you take charge of your life!

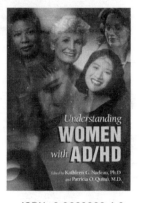

Understanding
WOMEN
with **AD/HD**
Edited by Kathleen G. Nadeau, Ph.D
and Patricia O. Quinn, M.D.

ISBN: 0-9660366-4-6
$19.95   468 pages

Order any of these exciting books
by phone, fax, or over the internet

ADVANTAGE BOOKS
1001 Spring Street, # 206

Silver Spring, MD 20910

888-238-8588 (toll free phone)

202-966-1561 (fax on demand)

Web Address: www.addvance.com
A Resource Site for Women and Girls with ADD

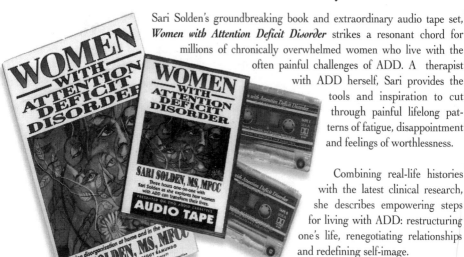

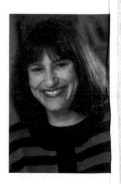
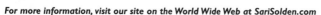